The International Behavioural and Social Sciences Library

MANAGERS

TAVISTOCK

INDUSTRIAL RELATIONS
In 13 Volumes

MANAGERS

Personality & Performance

KENN ROGERS

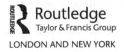

Routledge
Taylor & Francis Group

LONDON AND NEW YORK

First published in 1963 by
Tavistock Publications (1959) Limited

Published in 2001 by
Routledge
2 Park Square, Milton Park, Abingdon, Oxfordshire OX14 4RN
711 Third Avenue, New York, NY 10017

First issued in paperback 2014

Routledge is an imprint of the Taylor & Francis Group, an informa company

© 1963 Kenn Rogers

British Library Cataloguing in Publication Data
A CIP catalogue record for this book
is available from the British Library

Managers

Industrial Relations: 13 Volumes

The International Behavioural and Social Sciences Library
112 Volumes

ISBN 978-0-415-26446-4 (hbk)
ISBN 978-0-415-75359-3 (pbk)

Managers —
Personality &
Performance

KENN ROGERS

*First published in 1963
by Tavistock Publications (1959) Limited*

Contents

Contents

Acknowledgements

The writer wishes to thank the companies described here for their generosity in affording the use of their facilities and the time of their employees; also for their permission to record and cite the interviews. He also wishes to thank the respondents interviewed in the course of collecting the material for this study for their confidence and sympathy. Mr. J. M. M. Hill read through a draft of this book. The criticisms he has made were of great importance in rewriting the text.

I. What this book is about

In today's world the problem of economic growth is of concern to all. Why is it that some firms or industries develop and others stagnate; that some countries progress quickly while others remain backward or undeveloped? In seeking objective answers to such questions many, perhaps the majority, of studies proffer explanations that are based essentially upon the attributes of the environment in which the enterprise finds itself and concentrate attention upon such factors as the growth of demand, the lessening of taxes, the availability of capital, and the existence of mineral resources. These explanations do not take account of the *differential character* of individual firms and their *differential capacities* to cope with their environments whether favourable or unfavourable. Rather in the same way, we can, if we wish, explain the success or otherwise of an individual by reference to the opportunities existing for him, to his education, background, wealth. Such explanations neglect the individual himself and yet it is common experience that some individuals win out against most adverse circumstances while others fail with apparently every factor in their favour. Similarly, in a given economic climate and subject to the same broad economic conditions, one firm will succeed while another will fail. It is of interest to ask why this is so.

Such an inquiry is, of course, not based on the assumption that the environment does not matter. Clearly it does. Yet, in sheer practical reality there may be little a firm or, indeed, a country can do to alter the totality of its environment. Such changes tend to come slowly, usually as a result of

1

political action. There may, however, be more that can be done by paying attention to such factors as marketing policies and structures and manning of organizations which could prove more susceptible to change. Considerations of this kind are of special relevance to Britain, at present faced with the loss of many assets that acted in the past as a bulwark against economic storm. This will be of even greater importance if Britain enters a unifying supra-national trading area such as the Common Market, where the object will be to effect a 'harmonization', as the Rome Treaty has it, in such matters as tariffs, free movement of labour, payment for labour, social security, the result of which will be to reduce the differential environment that may now protect the less efficient. Particularly in these circumstances it is necessary to ask as objectively as one can: What leads to success for some firms and failure for others?, and to seek answers in terms of the quality of top-level management. For it is this group that decides the marketing policy of a company. In this context, marketing is seen as the 'creation and delivery of a standard of living' (McNair, 1961).

An examination of the literature dealing with the relationship between the quality of top-level management and economic growth produces meagre results. There is very little if anything in the nature of studies related to business success in other than purely economic terms and these are often unconvincing when examined as a guide to action. They tend to be anecdotal, written by business executives to support a series of beliefs. The reasons for this are many. Successful business men are not necessarily good at explaining their success, or at analysing it. Generally they are not trained investigators. As a result, what they write has some interest but it falls short of being a guide for the serious student of business. What these men really say is: 'Be like me and you'll be successful!' But what are these men like?

An analysis of these books shows that they describe the abilities and idiosyncrasies of these men. Frequently, they tend to ascribe their success to their idiosyncrasies and not to their abilities. The latter are often so deep-seated that the men themselves know very little about them. This is further enhanced by the social custom which frowns on talking about one's own abilities.

This separation of ability and mental make-up is also reinforced by a widely held belief that abilities are inborn and, therefore, one either has them or not. Mental attitudes, however, are seen as acquired, developed, and under one's conscious control. This viewpoint denies the existence of abilities which for emotional and often unconscious reasons may be deterred from coming into play.

Roy Lewis and Rosemary Stewart comment on the lack of studies related to top-level managers' psychological make-up in their book *The Boss* (1958). They call the business executive 'the man nobody knows'. According to them,

> . . . the psychologists have not been concerned with top management . . . there is almost nothing said about the lives, origins and inner thoughts of the men who control . . . a factory. . . . They do not suggest that at the top a man's own interest could ever conflict with his firm's; they do not deal with man as a political animal at all. If they suggest anything to the reader it is that life in business is simply plodding merit.

Officials of leading business organizations such as the Federation of British Industries, the Institute of Directors, the American Management Association and the National Association of Manufacturers assured the author in the course of his discussions with them that there were in fact no difficulties about the motivations of business executives. For example, one spokesman said: 'We always accept that

3

management is properly motivated.' When pressed about the meaning of 'properly', he defined it in terms of profits and company growth. After further discussion he made hesitant reference to two non-economic motives – status in terms of personal success and the desire to belong to a successful company.

This suggests that the valuation of executives' performances is generally viewed within a narrow framework of material rewards, security of employment, and, to a lesser degree, certain motives related to status. The theoretical possibility of other cultural, social, and psychological factors having an effect is often acknowledged, but in practice is usually fairly vigorously excluded from the general thinking. But this viewpoint begs the whole question of how a man becomes a successful businessman and why he wants to be one. It has often been shown that workers are influenced by many factors other than their rates of pay and security of employment. Up to now, however, it has not been widely accepted that this is true also for managers. One reason for this is that such studies as are undertaken in industry tend to be paid for by management, and it is a general observation that human beings tend to dislike self-examination, particularly when this involves an examination of their motives.

Business executives, like all human beings, respond to complex motivational patterns which are shaped by biological and environmental forces. The necessities of business may superimpose modifications on the existing motivation pattern of an executive, and it may well be that the success or failure of a business organization is intimately linked to the capacity of its executives to adjust themselves to a given business reality. It is, however, a bold assumption that these realities are the sole guide to the behaviour of business executives when engaged in their corporate activities. If it is the capacity to adjust which tips the scales between success and failure, it

4

becomes important to examine the conditions that help or hinder such adjustment.

Katona (1951) has pointed to the need to examine economic behaviour in a wider frame than economics only. He states that:

'. . . economic processes stem directly from human behaviour and . . . this simple but important fact has not received its due in modern economic analysis . . . resources from both economics and psychology need to be used to arrive at a realistic analysis of economic behaviour.'

It follows from this that the analysis of economic behaviour requires concepts drawn from social sciences other than economics. One economist who appears to have followed this up is Barna (1961), who, in an unpublished report to the European Productivity Agency, comments:

'The character of a firm is determined by its management . . . In almost all firms the different manifestations of the firm's behaviour – price policy, marketing policy, inventory policy, labour policy, investment policy – are just different aspects of the management's character.'

If this is correct, then business activity must be viewed, as, indeed, must all human behaviour, as designed to satisfy not only the obvious rational economic purposes but also emotional needs, both overt and recondite, some of which may be healthy and others neurotic in character. In this century clinical psychology has gone some way to show that the part of the mind of which we are ordinarily not aware, the unconscious, influences much that we think or do. Often the true motives beneath our behaviour are hidden from us, so that despite the utmost conscious 'sincerity' desires of which we are totally unaware play a strong part in determining our behaviour. Clearly, the decisions of senior executives affect the operation of entire organizations. These decisions, however, are in turn affected by the way the various members of the firm perceive their own work, the function of the organization, its business purpose, and the reason for which the company has been set up. Bion (1961) examined the behaviour of groups and their capacity to deal effectively with their tasks. He used an approach which combined the concepts of psycho-analysis focused on the individual with those of group dynamics, which, through their special concepts, reveal different aspects of the same phenomena. He particularly studied the basic idea of a group which has a task, and the factors which interfere with carrying out this task as planned. This can be illustrated by several observations.

One might be that of a psychotic person who cannot perform even the simplest task necessary for his own survival, such as feeding or cleaning himself. Others can be related to neurotics. They may be hampered in achieving success in marriage, hobbies, or work by the existence of emotional factors. The neurotic may well conceive how the task is to be done, but emotional factors may deter him. Quite often this means that the task itself has taken on certain symbolic and unknown values to which the failure can be traced. For example, the individual who wants to succeed in an examination or in getting a particular job may surprisingly fail to do so, although his ability for the task is more than adequate. Upon analysis it might be found that accomplishing the task represents unconsciously a triumph over the father or a sibling. If this is not known to the individual, it may lead to deep feelings of anxiety, guilt, fear of retributive attacks by the father or sibling, and in some instances to failure in achieving the set task. Neurotic behaviour in this sense means that past conflicts are unconsciously repeated by the individual and projected into

6

situations or on to people to whom they are not related. By contrast the so-called normal person may also have problems of the kind ascribed to the neurotic. They can, however, be controlled. Either their intensity is not so great that they seriously affect behaviour or the individual may be aware of their nature and thereby be in a position effectively to control his action.

When these clinical observations are extended to business executives, all kinds of behaviour, which on the face of it may appear contradictory or at least difficult to explain, can become a good deal clearer. When a business decision, viewed in the light of economic factors, appears to be illogical, it is quite likely to be comprehensible in the context of the psychological make-up of the people who make the decision.

The objective task to be carried out, whether it is running a factory or marketing a particular product, will simultaneously have both an overt and a symbolic meaning. Unless this symbolic meaning, that is, the appreciation of the work at an unconscious fantasy level, broadly corresponds to that in the individual's consciousness, the individual is heading for difficulties, inefficiency, and potential failure. In such instances, the conscious and the unconscious of the individual work in opposite directions and hence against each other. Consciously, the individual may want to do one thing; unconsciously, he may desire something different.

These concepts make work, regardless of its specific nature, subject to analysis of a far greater subtlety than is usually perceived. The average working day, as well as the structure of the average job, provides for the individual a whole host of different experiences and opportunities to live out his emotional life. Obviously, the kind of work the individual does and the work of the organization in which he occupies a role are most important determinants.

One quite general observation may be made at this point.

All firms exist and survive solely on the basis of an interchange with their environment, exporting something from themselves to the outside world and importing something in exchange. To put it simply – they trade. This means that there must be objects outside them that need their products and services and on which they are dependent for survival. This is true not only for firms but for human life itself, and such dependence on external figures characterizes especially the life of the infant and sets up from the start of life – conflict. There is conflict in attitudes to these external figures that are both valued for their capacity to give and hated for their equal capacity to withhold. One focus of examination must therefore be the attitude of the senior executive to his market and to the symbolic importance of those outside him in the market whom he 'services' with his products.

The way in which such attitudes manifest themselves may be considered in relation to three case histories, which though anecdotal may nevertheless serve to illustrate how attitudes to the ultimate consumer influence economic decision-taking.

CASE HISTORY I

A large European company engaged in renting domestic equipment experienced an appreciable drop in market share relative to its competitors, although its business volume was increasing and its profits were substantial. Internal analysis of the company showed that a good flow of new business was largely offset by a large number of cancellations from subscribers. A survey commissioned to determine the causes for this found the fault to lie in the relationship between the company and its subscribers. Only in exceptional circumstances were complaints related to the quality of the company's service. However, the manner in which they were handled left a great deal to be desired.

The company on going into business rented out radio sets only. It was reluctant to introduce television sets and did not do so until many years later. This was so, in spite of the fact that television had been widely accepted by the public and the company's competitors had actively exploited the opportunites in this market for many years. The company had decided on a sales policy according to which its customers could rent only a radio receiver, but were not able to subscribe to television alone. If they wanted a television set, subscribers had to accept both. This was a practice in marked contrast to the demand of the market and to all its competitors' policies.

Market research revealed that the company's personnel were seen as efficient but unfriendly, and even arrogant. Collectors were often short-tempered. The equipment was invariably described by subscribers as good or excellent in performance but often shabby in appearance. The company's showrooms, which also served as collection centres, lacked chairs for the public. This was rationalized as a deliberate policy – 'to keep them [the customers] moving'. In recorded group interviews, when these and other complaints were voiced by present and past subscribers, the general tenor was succinctly expressed by one participant when stating 'They do not want our business. Look at the Board [of Directors]. Among them are the lords of our country. They look down on us and think they are doing us a favour.' When this recording was played back to a high-level manager of the company, he exclaimed: 'But they have no right to complain!'

CASE HISTORY II

An African grain-milling company, although protected by government-regulated import and production quotas, experienced increasing pressure from its smaller competitors.

Changes in the sales force, channels of distribution, and advertising failed to produce more business. Although market analysis showed a strong consumer preference for bread bought retail over the traditional native-made flour meal, the latter remained the mainstay of the company's activities. The Board of Directors strongly resisted suggestions that it should start bakeries. One Board member went so far as to state: 'Do you realize that if today you'll give them bread, tomorrow they'll want shoes, the next day independence!'

When the company's trade symbol was presented for testing purposes, only a few respondents among a sample of several hundred recognized it. This was the more surprising as the company had used this symbol extensively for many years. It turned out that the trade symbol represented something widely known in the Western world but neither known nor found in the company's business territory, which extended across an area of about one thousand miles. It had been designed in Europe. Its colour composition had been tested for African climatic conditions. It was, however, not considered necessary to check it for recognition by Africans.

CASE HISTORY III

A major American banking organization transferred several of its branch offices to a competitive institution for a price that no more than covered the cost of the premises' leases. The reason for this action stated at the time was that the original owner of the branches did not see any profit for itself in that retail banking operation. It is alleged that in a less formal manner a member of its top-level management expressed himself by saying: 'I cannot see how it could pay us to have these people come *trampling* into our branches.' Several years later, a new management team greatly deplored the loss of these branches. Its competitor seemed able to make a success of retail banking in branches. Indeed, in accordance with America's strict banking laws, branches represent one of the limited number of avenues along which banking business activities can be expanded. The interesting feature of this bank's operation was that its avowed policy was to expand into retail banking, which in general was found to be a highly profitable sector. Yet, when it had the opportunity to put this policy into action, its management displayed a marked reluctance to do so.

Common factors in each of these three cases were:

1. The companies were big and had therefore grown in the past.
2. Their markets were changing against the background of broader political and cultural development.
3. They preferred to rely in the conduct of their business largely on their economic strength, while using modern marketing only marginally.
4. Their actual products and services differed only slightly from those of competitors.
5. They had competitors organized similarly to themselves to whom they lost market shares.
6. Their top-level managements seemed to be more interested in social superiority than in a healthy and expanding business.

Everything thus seemed to favour the continued development of these firms, except the attitudes of their senior executives, which were characterized by contempt for and isolation from their market. The suggestion, therefore, arises that different attitudes could have produced different results in terms of economic growth. Yet to examine this fully requires the discovery of several firms with differential degrees of success in the same market and the opportunity

11

to study attitudes of executives in both the successful and the less successful firms within this market. This book is about such an opportunity and the results of such a study.

It examines the problem of economic growth in terms of the rise to prominence over a relatively short period of time of a firm in an industry with a stable pattern of distribution, and compares this with other firms that did not grow. The book is not in any sense intended as a success story nor does it delineate or advocate formulas for business progress. Instead it is concerned with the pattern of progress in the industry described, with the contrast between the dynamic and the less dynamic, the successful and the stagnating. This it seeks to explain in a relatively novel way not merely in terms of economic forces, market needs, and competitive pressures but also in terms of the personalities of the men in charge of companies, their enthusiasms and hesitations, their attitudes of mind and the origins of these attitudes.

When examining a business organization what one essentially does is look at a group of people gathered for a 'common purpose'. It has been stated before that the motives of the various members of such a group are not necessarily identical among themselves or with those of the firm itself. Although there may be differences between the motivations of the various members, both in nature and in degree, all co-operate towards the common purpose of the group. This act of co-operation is common to members of the organization and is vital for its survival (Barnard, 1956). The success in accomplishing this purpose can be assessed by the degree to which members have been able to achieve their task while simultaneously adapting themselves to the demands of their environment, both external and internal, and thereby assuring the continuity of the operation. In this sense, the way in which a group organizes itself, i.e. the structure of a company, represents an expression of the strategy it uses

WHAT THIS BOOK IS ABOUT

while carrying out its task (Argyris, 1959). Another expression of its strategy is its marketing plan. Here, marketing is seen to embrace all the activities of a company, from recognizing consumers' needs, through expressing those needs into specifications for production of products and services, to delivering them to consumers in a manner desired by them and profitable to the company. The use of skills by members of the organization when carrying out their task can then be seen as tactics within the strategy.

It has been suggested above that an organization's results are affected by the interaction of its members among themselves and between the group as a whole and its external environment, e.g. its market (the users of its products and services), its trade (its immediate buyers), its competitors, the government of the country in which it operates and its laws. From this two main questions arise:

What affects these interactions? and
What affects the individuals' use of their skills in a positive way and what interferes with it?

To answer these questions the major hypotheses of this study have been formulated. They are:

(i) It is to be generally assumed that the ability to perceive a business situation creatively, the most important quality of managers, is directly related to their ability alternately to identify with the people in the situation, e.g. trade customers, consumers, workers, shareholders, competitors, public opinion, and to return to their own and their companies' environment without experiencing unbearable anxieties in the process. Unbearable anxieties, depending upon their intensity will invoke defences leading to neurotic inefficiency and in the extreme to psychotic disintegration. In an industrial organization, however, as

13

indeed in life, adjustment to total reality is a factor of success.

More specifically it is assumed that:

(ii) The success of a company's business operations, measured by profits and, even more, by its share of the market, is directly affected by the attitudes of its top-level executives towards both products and consumers. Other things being equal, these attitudes, sometimes conscious but often unconscious, will have a major effect on the company's business success.

(iii) The underlying attitudes of those in command of a company may at times conflict with the overt business policy of the company. Such a situation creates a stress condition which will affect the company adversely.

(iv) The rank and file of a company as well as its consultants, researchers, and advertising agents tend to align their perception of the consumer and the product with that adopted by the company's top-level executives. This process seems to be facilitated by a tendency on the part of management to hire staff 'in its own image'.

II. The research opportunity

Ideally, the best method when attempting to examine a business organization would be to adopt the same procedure as the scientist does in the laboratory. He holds all the variables in an experiment constant except one. Obviously, business life is far too complicated to permit this to be done. The only alternative, therefore, is to select an industry where as many variables as possible happen to be constant. This is much easier said than done. Preliminary examination caused the author to rule out such industries as steel, food processing, and textiles. But manufacturers of household products seemed to present a fruitful area of study. On the one hand, these products designed to lighten domestic chores were increasingly coming to the fore and were increasingly accepted as necessities in the 'affluent society'. That is to say, they were indicative of pronounced growth characteristics. On the other hand, firms making these household products were usually part of an industrial combine which also manufactured a range of industrial and other capital goods. Broad characteristics of these household products were as follows:

(i) There was an extensive similarity among models in the various product groups. This was expressed in the following:

(a) As far as price, performance, quality, style, and appearance were concerned, brands were almost standardized (see page 32).

(b) The system of distribution in this sector of the industry was highly uniform, and one large

15

national chain in particular sold by far the largest aggregate volume of this type of product (see page 32).

(ii) Analyses of the market revealed that in most of the product groups, one, two, or three companies, from now on called 'leaders', held nearly one-half to two-thirds of the market, while the rest, from now on called 'non-leaders', was divided among between twelve and thirty-two firms (see *Table 1*, p. 17). Moreover, about 10 per cent of the companies, the leaders, supplied more than half of the total market, while about 90 per cent of the companies, the non-leaders, supplied less than half of the market. These analyses made by commercial research firms, tallying reasonably well with those of governmental organizations, gave fairly accurate and detailed statistical information about ownership among the various consumer groups, as well as about market patterns in these product groups.

(iii) The size of a company and its financial resources did not seem to have any bearing on its market position in this industry. Companies holding a small share in this market ranged from the smallest (sales equivalent to several hundred thousand dollars in household products annually) to the largest (total sales of every type of product in this industry to the equivalent of several hundred million dollars annually).

(iv) External conditions, such as government-imposed credit restrictions, instalment purchase regulations, sales taxes, level of general employment, and income redistribution, seemed to have affected the entire industry equally.

(v) The industry was generally recognized as one of the key areas of economic growth. In one year, when this study was conducted, its household products represented, at the retail level, nearly 1½ per cent of the total national product (GNP) in the country. Whenever instalment purchase regulations were either imposed or eased, this product group was one of the most affected.

(vi) For many years managements were remarkably alike, until one firm broke with tradition by bringing in a management team from outside the industry. The

TABLE 1. MANUFACTURERS' PRODUCTS FOUND IN HOMES, SHOWING DISTRIBUTION OF MARKET SHARES*

		Leaders in the Market		All other Manufacturers		
			Market shares	Number of	Market shares	
Product groups	Number of Leaders	1952–1956	1954–1958	Manufac-turers	1952–1956	1954–1958
		%	%		%	%
A	3	54·3	52·2	14	45·7	47·8
B	2	61·4	60·7	27	38·6	39·3
C	3	63·7	55·4	12	36·3	44·6
D	1	57·8	63·2	22	42·2	36·8
E	1	57·7	65·8	32	42·3	34·2
F	3	45·8	68·9	16	54·2	31·1
G	2	56·3	59·1	31	43·7	40·9
H	2	58·8	54·6	29	41·2	45·4
I	2	54·4	70·2	14	46·6	29·8
J	3	49·5	N.A.	11	50·5	N.A.
Total Average	2·2	56·0	61·1	20·8	44·0	38·9
Total number of companies involved	14			123		

*At the request of the firms studied, it has been necessary to eliminate specific references to them as well as to the products. The selection of the material and particularly the form of its presentation were guided by these requests.

introduction of this one variable into what was otherwise a quasi-equilibrium provided an unusual opportunity for the study of an industry in almost laboratory conditions. It is the basis for this study.

This company, in this study called Universal, has a division which manufactures and sells household products. In 1955–56 its turnover represented less than 3 per cent of the total business of the company and it sustained a very considerable loss. By 1959 this division's contribution to Universal's total volume of business came to more than 7 per cent and it added a substantial portion to its total profits. In 1955 the division was manufacturing more than twenty different types of products and its share of the total market was less than 5 per cent. By 1959, concentrating its efforts on a limited number of products, it had reached a commanding position in the market for them.

This transformation is sufficiently notable to command closer attention. The achievement is even more striking when placed in the context of the industry as a whole, for, while Universal's household product division was enjoying this large measure of success its competitors, with similar products and opportunities, failed to make comparable progress.

The study described here was divided into three parts. First, a study of the market conditions in the industry going back in time more generally about twenty-five years and more specifically about seven to ten years was carried out. The former related to estimates of production, and to the patterns of distribution, pricing, and diversification of models in the ten product groups selected for analysis in the industry. The latter was in terms of market shares, ownership of the products by consumers, patterns of distribution, product development, the organizational structures of several companies, and details on the business background of a number of high-level executives manning these structures. Second, a comprehensive pilot study extending over nearly two years was carried out. In the course of this work nine manufacturing companies were contacted. Five of them co-operated in the full programme. They belonged to the group of non-leaders in the industry. In addition, editors of trade journals, research organizations, advertising agents, wholesale and retail outlets, as well as housewife consumers, were included. The study reached from the boardroom to the departments concerned with design, production, advertising, and marketing, and to the sales and shipping floor at both wholesale and retail level. It involved nearly three hundred people.

One particular difficulty assails anyone making a study of an industry, whether it is intended to be descriptive or analytic. In assembling the material the co-operation of many leading figures in the industry becomes essential. If it is published in exactly its original form it is liable to cause embarassment and hostility. While many people are prepared to talk freely, only the explicit understanding that their confidences will be respected will induce them to do so. On the other hand, if the description of the study is tampered with or omissions are made, then the work is no longer a scientific document. To overcome this dilemma one concession had to be made to the feelings of those who are portrayed herein, sometimes unflatteringly. Every description and every quotation appears in the form in which it was originally made, but the names of individuals and companies are either withheld or changed. The country in which this study was carried out, one of the major Western industrialized nations, is deliberately left vague. The study is described as relating to an industry with a very wide range of products, but, again, their specific nature has been deliberately left vague. The reader is assured that beyond this no other changes have been made.

All the individuals who appear in these pages have been given the opportunity to pass judgement on the study. Few – very few – have agreed with its conclusions. Moreover, even they declared their assent with varying degrees of strength. The great majority declined to express a view on the grounds that they did not feel themselves qualified to do so. A small minority revealed vehement hostility, some going so far as to call it nonsense. Some brought forth their own explanations, ascribing success or failure in the industry to management training, a particular pattern of organization, or the entry of outsiders into a hitherto closely knit group of firms. Each of these explanations is interesting in itself and may not be without some validity. I hope, however, that it will soon become clear that in this particular instance, at least, a further and more fundamental factor must be taken into account – the psychology of those whose role it is to make the key decisions about the various aims and policies of companies.

To carry out a study of the kind outlined in the previous chapter depends always on the consent of the people concerned. To obtain that consent the wishes and apprehensions of the individuals as well as the conditions generally prevailing in the particular industry must be fully considered. Some of the former, especially the desire to remain anonymous and its effects on the presentation of the material, have already been mentioned. There is also another problem to be faced: people are unlikely to talk freely about their innermost feelings and thoughts. If they are ordered to do so, as in the course of this study higher-level managers of one company attempted to do with their subordinates, this merely increases anxiety and tends to make the task of the researcher more difficult. One of the major instruments employed in this kind of work is the skill of the researcher, not only when analysing socio-economic conditions affecting an industry but even more so when observing or interviewing people. This is his capacity to pick up and interpret the moods and feelings prevailing in a given situation, his ability to comprehend the attitude of respondents: what they really want to communicate and frequently what they try to withhold.

In addition to direct observation and interviews, there are tools in the form of tests available for this kind of work. Those employed in one part of this study are described in greater detail in Appendix A. However, the diagnostic and predictive value of any psychological test depends heavily on the various psychological and social forces affecting the respondent when the test takes place. Experience in the pilot study showed that the use of such devices as psychological tests gave rise to fears and anxieties in the individuals concerned. This is doubly unfortunate. Not only does it unsettle the respondent; often he fears – and no amount of reassurance seems adequate to allay this fear – that the results of these tests may be reported to his superiors in the company. On top of all this is a natural and inevitable fear that he may 'fail' the test. No explanation that these devices are merely stimulants and there is no question of either success or failure can wholly overcome this anxiety. If, as sometimes happens, he discusses these worries with his colleagues at the time of the test or subsequently, then feelings of hostility spread throughout the section of the company concerned, which makes the task of the researcher even harder. There is also an element of unfairness in arousing anxiety in these individuals, particularly about their jobs – even more so in view of their co-operation in the study. Moreover, people feel with some justification that such tests have as an aim the extraction from them of information of which they are not aware – a form of stealing.

21

It is true that the use of tests can facilitate quantification, though it is not always clear what is being quantified. Psychological test data represent subjective judgements arrived at by application of arbitrarily set standards. They assess effects related to psychological dimensions by unknown laws. For example, we may wish to measure a man's ability but we can only gauge its effects that bear an undetermined relation to it (Stevens, 1951). That is to say, he may at a point in time be unable to use his full ability because of emotional reasons such as anxiety in the testing situation, or he may be unwilling to use his full ability for conscious reasons such as the knowledge that 'high test scores' will prevent him from getting a job while 'lower test scores' will qualify him. The latter, of course, makes greater use of his abilities than the former by consciously manipulating the overt effects of his ability towards a lower level of performance. The test results, however, may indicate this manoeuvre only to an exceptionally skilled and insightful tester. The reader to whom this sounds improbable is referred to Whyte's *The Organization Man* (1956), where this is described and discussed in great detail. Consequently, these projective devices, although often immensely useful in indicating a person's attitudes, do not provide conclusive evidence. Finally, the author took the view that quantification by itself is not necessarily a virtue and that it was more important to attempt to provide a setting in which the real perceptions and motivations of those concerned could emerge and be observed and studied in as unobstructed a way as possible. In view of these considerations, the author mainly relied in this study on the interview as his most important research tool.

Statistical methods were employed in the economic analysis of conditions prevailing in the industry, particularly relating to market shares and advertising expenditures.

When they were used in the analysis of the developmental background of Universal's executives, they promptly showed their limitations, especially in the fact that it was impossible to obtain the necessary data from all the members in the group.

Another important factor in this kind of work is money. The conditions prevailing in the country when this research was carried out precluded large-scale studies to a considerable degree; the necessary funds were simply not available. Consequently, it depended greatly on having a researcher who happened to have enough money and the desire to undertake research into some of the causes of business success and failure. The author was fortunate in being able to meet both requirements. Limiting though this is, it is not without advantage. People tend to get to know an individual and form a relationship of confidence with him; to maintain the same relationship with a group of investigators or even with a particular research institute might be more difficult.

Very little overt resistance on the part of the interviewees was experienced by the researcher. Of the nine companies contacted, five, all non-leaders, co-operated to the fullest extent, though in releasing the material for publication they eliminated a great deal of what they considered 'personal'. Two leader companies contacted during this stage offered co-operation. One even invited it in writing. However, both, shortly after reading the transcripts of their initial interviews, suggested that further research, at least among higher-level executives, should be carried out in the form of questions submitted by the author in writing, which they then offered to answer in writing. Clearly, this procedure would not have proved fruitful, except possibly to demonstrate resistance to the study. At Universal, among eighty-seven respondents, the researcher encountered only four who showed anxiety to a degree that would have made further contact unproductive.

Two reasons may account for the friendly and co-operative attitude displayed. One was the fact that the author, being a foreigner, more particularly a transient, did not represent a general threat to the interviewees, who, feeling safe, could communicate more or less freely. The other was that the author, though introduced as a psychologist, was known to have been active in business, particularly to have 'met a payroll'. This afforded him *a priori* the mark of 'business experience plus'. It sometimes seemed that the interviewees in fact welcomed the opportunity of discussing their business problems with a neutral outsider, particularly one who could speak their own business language.

Each interview was started off by stating the full purpose of the study. Professional confidence was assured at all times. At the end of each interview the author offered to answer to the best of his ability any questions the respondent wished to ask. Significantly, many respondents made inquiries of a highly personal nature. This can be interpreted as a form of retaliation. There was, however, in several instances a rather naïve search for a simple success formula which 'surely the author should have'. Many times, the author was pumped for information about competitors and even colleagues in the same firm. Consciously or unconsciously, these questions represented tests as to whether he actually was or would remain discreet.

Two precautions in particular were observed. In the first place care was taken throughout the study not to give the interviewees any indication of the author's interpretations of the material provided by them. The research study, it must be remembered, was an attempt to observe and not to effect changes. Second, every effort was made to recognize and allow for the possible distorting effects his own emotional attitudes might have on his perception and interpretation of the material. The kind of danger of which he had to beware

24

was of allowing a liking or dislike for any particular person to cause him unconsciously to adopt or reject that person's viewpoint. During the period of the study he underwent intensive personal psycho-analysis and thus was able to find an objective point of reference for his own attitudes.

In one particular, carrying out this study did affect the author's own attitudes. It brought home to him the importance of respecting the people with whom he worked, regardless of the attitudes they themselves displayed. For example, one business executive may well express his anxieties and unconscious resistance in the form of an emphasis on his self-importance. Another may display apparent inefficiency to a considerable degree. It is essential in such circumstances neither to accept the first executive's own valuation of himself nor to fall into the opposite trap of feeling superior to the second.

The work with members of the five companies yielded a wealth of relevant material, but the use that could be made of it was limited, owing to the need to gain agreement to its publication by the executives of the companies concerned. Before work commenced with any member of a company, he was informed that the purpose of the study was to find the reasons for the distributional structure of the industry's market as detailed in *Table 1*.

When the pilot study had been completed, a much more detailed and intensive examination of one single firm was undertaken – the household products division of Universal. This organization, as indicated in the introduction, is unusual in that a management team from outside the industry had been introduced. Moreover, while it was not among the leaders at that time, it was clearly improving its position in a striking fashion. Transition from non-leader to leader in an industry is sufficiently unusual to warrant further study. Having selected this company, the author focused attention upon the following factors, which provided a framework for his interviews and observations.

1. Why did the management of this company change?
2. Why were new men from outside the industry selected?
3. What changes did the new executives institute?
4. What motivated these changes?
5. How did these changes affect the activity of the company?
6. How did these changes affect the trading position of the company?
7. Did the company's recent marketing efforts help to broaden the total market for these products?
8. How did these executives view:
    (*a*) their products,
    (*b*) their markets,
    (*c*) their jobs,
    (*d*) their company,
    (*e*) their competitors in the industry?
9. What was the relationship of these executives to their own background?
10. What did these executives expect from the future?

As in the pilot study, the investigation extended throughout the hierarchy of the company from its sales force, service organization, and packing departments to the boardroom. A total of eighty-seven men and women were interviewed; they were mainly members of the company, but a few were from its advertising agency. Some of the company's employees were interviewed as often as five times. The interviews lasted from forty minutes to three hours. A special arrangement was made with the managing director, Mr. Alexander. A total of at least thirty hours was spent with him. In addition to a series of interviews, the author was allowed to sit in his office while normal business was conducted, and this over extended periods of time. It was also found possible to accompany him on a business trip to his factory. There were further opportunities for contact with senior executives and salesmen outside their own offices.

If the concepts stated in Chapter I were valid, it was reasonable to assume that, in the household product industry selected for this study, the attitudes among executives towards their work might vary to a considerable degree. They might depend on who these men considered the consumer to be, that is to say who was to be serviced and satisfied. One factor in this situation would be the needs of the housewife; another, the wish of the executive to satisfy these needs. By themselves, these two factors represent a fairly straightforward situation. Their unconscious meanings, however, make them potentially far more complex. The wish to satisfy the housewife's needs can, for example, be closely associated with unresolved wishes to replace the husband, and, in so far as the housewife is unconsciously standing for the mother, hence to replace the father. Depending, then, on the amount of triumph or failure in relation to the father in the individual's mind, this would represent a bi-polar situation of potentially dangerous or healthy competition. This, of course, is only one example. It is not unreasonable to assume that expressions of these attitudes will vary among executives in successful and less successful companies. More specifically, they might manifest themselves in the ability of these men to identify with the housewife and also in general attitudes towards such identification, that is to say, giving a service to these housewives. Moreover, it is not unlikely that some executives might perceive the housewife as an intruder who judges their efforts in a negative way, i.e. she will not admit their value. Clearly, such an attitude, whether held consciously or unconsciously,

27

is not conducive to confidence when making business decisions. If, however, the housewife can be seen as able to be satisfied and to respond with gratitude, i.e. to be likely to buy the products, this would potentially give greater confidence to the executive when making the necessary business decisions, though in so far as her satisfaction was felt to represent a triumph over father, guilt would thereby be increased.

The hypothesis stated in Chapter I should therefore be illustrated by the following observations:

(i) The attitudes of executives in the household product sector of this industry towards their markets are affected by the ease with which they identify themselves with the female roles in the use of these products, e.g. cleaning, preparing food, washing. The less anxiety it causes these executives to identify with these female roles, the more positive will be their attitude towards their consumers and, consequently, the more positively will they attempt to stimulate and satisfy the needs of housewives for these products.

(ii) The attitudes of these executives towards their products are affected by the two main functions which household products perform for housewives. They serve to lighten household chores and they are symbols of social and economic well-being.

III. Significant features of the household product market

An analysis of general conditions in this household product market pointed to four features that were particularly relevant to this study. They were:

1. Household products as symbols of social and economic well-being.
2. The growth of the working-class market.
3. The high degree of similarity between the products of the various manufacturers.
4. The pattern of distribution of the industry's products.

HOUSEHOLD PRODUCTS – SYMBOLS OF SOCIAL AND ECONOMIC WELL-BEING

There is little doubt that in the country in which this study was conducted, as indeed in many parts of the world, ownership of household products is widely regarded as a symbol of superior standards of living. Pride of ownership, the feeling of economic well-being, even the keen, if 'unworthy' pleasure of 'keeping up with the Joneses', all these things, as the writers of advertisements have long recognized, can enhance the desire to buy them.

One particular aspect of 'keeping up with the Joneses' needs to be mentioned here. There is a very general desire among women to liberate themselves from what they are coming to regard as drudgery. This finds expression in the emergence of an increasing feeling of dissatisfaction on the part of the ordinary housewife with the restricting range of her house-hold duties, particularly the more menial ones. It also arises from the feeling that her efforts cannot be adequately appreciated, since at the end of a day's exhausting work she has little to show. The effect of this is threefold. First, there is an emotional need to lighten the burden of housework. Second, there is a tendency to find work outside the home, not only for financial but also for social and emotional reasons. Third, there has been a very great drop in the number of women prepared to go into domestic service.

These factors would in themselves create a lively potential market for household products. But their impact is magnified when the social pressures mentioned earlier are taken into account. A woman who might in other circumstances be quite content to carry out her role as a housewife observes her neighbours with their burden of work apparently lightened and becomes dissatisfied if she herself is denied the means of following suit.

THE GROWTH OF THE WORKING-CLASS MARKET

The most significant single development in the market for consumer goods of all kinds over the last twenty years has been the growth of working-class prosperity during and after the second world war. It is due to a number of factors of which the most important is full employment; to maintain this is now accepted as a major obligation of government. Other factors that have operated to increase working-class prosperity are the redistribution of income that has taken place during this period, the introduction of measures of social security, and the fact that so many working-class families have more than one, perhaps two or even three, wage-earners. This has created a market for consumer goods that is numerically large. Moreover, the impact of these changes has been reinforced by the difference between middle-class and working-class patterns of expenditure.

The middle-class family traditionally accepts heavy social and family calls upon its purse. School fees, mortgage payments, holidays away from home, greater expenditure on clothes, the cost of running a car, are all claims which bite into the family's budget. The working-class family is much more likely to be living in housing accommodation owned by a municipality or a rent-controlled dwelling rented from a private landlord. It spends considerably less money on education or on improving property. As a result, a working-class family with several wage-earners may well have more free spending money than a middle-class family with one wage-earner receiving the same gross pay, since taxation on one large income is larger than on a number of small ones.

It is reasonable to conjecture – though direct evidence is lacking – that, in general, the working-class family has comparatively little tradition of thrift. This may arise from the fact that its spending habits were in many cases formed at a time when there was little or nothing to save. As a result, working-class thrift has generally tended to be directed into certain narrow channels, such as small industrial insurance policies. Even today, in a time of much greater prosperity, the working-class propensity to save is much smaller than that of the middle or upper income groups. The government, trying to damp down the demand for consumer goods, implicitly recognizes this in its policy of restricting instalment buying by the imposition of minimum deposits; families that are able to make repayment of the equivalent of a few dollars apparently find great difficulty in saving a larger amount required as a deposit.

This can be explained in psychological terms. People who have been deprived will tend to insist upon immediate gratification of their desires when the opportunity permits. They

31

are much less likely to be prepared to postpone immediate satisfaction in order to enjoy a greater benefit later on.

PRODUCT SIMILARITY

For most household products, there is comparatively little product differential between different makes and different manufacturers. All look very much alike, perform alike, and, for a given type or size, are sold at roughly the same price through the same channels of distribution.

What in most instances appears to have happened is this. Some companies developed and marketed household products designed to ease the housewives' chores. Competing manufacturers were quick to follow these leads. But with few exceptions these manufacturers did not go out into the field to investigate the market. They assumed from the statements of wholesalers that the successful competitors knew what they were doing and that consumer acceptance of a product is evidence of satisfaction with it. They did not question whether such assumed consumer satisfaction might only be relative to the offerings of competition. They accepted consumer preference as tantamount to consumer satisfaction.

THE PATTERN OF DISTRIBUTION

This product similarity is interesting on two counts. In the first place, it might be expected to lead to a fairly regular distribution of market shares. Even if historical advantage or other factors had acted to put one firm in a dominant position in a particular product group and thus give it the largest market share, it could reasonably be expected that at least some of its competitors would have substantial shares of the market. Even the textbook oligopolistic

32

situation assumes that the few firms that are competing divide the market between them with some degree of symmetry.

However, in the various product groups there are one, two, or three companies which supply more than half of the market, while the rest of the manufacturers, averaging about 21 in number, splinter the balance of the market among themselves (see *Table 1*). Their average market share is about 2 per cent. There are at least 137 companies engaged in manufacture in the ten product groups listed in *Table 1*, many among them multi-product companies. There are 14 market leaders, among them, also, multi-product firms. This indicates that about 10 per cent of the manufacturers, the leaders, supply rather more than half of the market, while all the rest (90 per cent) of the manufacturers supply less than half. It also seems that the leaders in each product group maintain their lead and this, on the whole, in increasing measure. (The figures for the two five-year periods overlap by about two and a half years, which makes it difficult to assess this trend more exactly.)

Second, it is significant that there does not seem to be a correlation between the absolute size of a company measured by its capital, its assets, or its total sales volume and its share of the market. Companies which have a toehold in a given household product market range from those whose total sales amount to the equivalent of a few hundred thousand dollars per annum to those whose total sales are in excess of several hundred million dollars annually. The leading companies in the various household product groups are not the giants but the small and medium companies in this industry. Nor is the market share of a company, as will be seen later, related to advertising expenditure (see *Figures 1* and *2*, pp. 86, 87).

IV. The non-leader companies

During the course of the pilot study detailed material was gathered from personnel of the non-leader companies, that is, those which, as has been shown, have consistently only very small market shares. Salesmen, buyers, demonstrators, and retail customers were interviewed. Some salesmen were accompanied on their daily calls. Use was also made of projective devices such as Sentence Completion, Rosenzweig P–F cartoons, and TAT-type sketches.

Interviews were also held with executives of these companies. It proved impossible, however, to gain their co-operation in the use of projective devices; though they would gladly co-operate in arranging for projective tests of their sales staff, they refused without exception to participate in them themselves. However, the series of personal interviews with non-leader executives provided an adequately clear picture of their attitudes.

From the material gathered as the pilot study proceeded, it became possible to build two composite profiles, one of executives, the other of salesmen, all employed by non-leader companies. It quickly became apparent that there was a close relationship between the attitudes of the executives and the salesmen to the extent that they seemed to mirror each other.

PROFILE OF NON-LEADER EXECUTIVES

Dealing first with the attitudes of non-leader executives, as they evolved from this series of interviews, their attitudes

34

to their products and their consumers can be illustrated under seven headings.

- (a) Their companies' distributors, i.e. wholesalers, multiples, dealers.
- (b) The various sectors of their companies, i.e. marketing, product-planning, advertising, selling, service.
- (c) The household products.
- (d) The consumer.
- (e) Government policies and regulations.
- (f) Their successful competitors.
- (g) Their own business activities.

(a) Attitudes to Distributors

Manufacturers of these household products distribute their goods through wholesalers, multiples, smaller dealers and to consumers directly, either in combination with dealers or without them. Fairly early in each interview the question was posed to executives: 'To whom do you sell your products?' One answered:

'To whom do we sell? Mostly wholesalers, that is to say, they take the larger portion of our production. Only a lesser quantity goes to retail outlets, multiples, etc. We have often considered broadening our base and shifting more of the distribution directly to retailers. But so far we are not successful in this. At least not as much as we would like to be. It is difficult to do this. There are the wholesalers to be considered, and there are our various other outlets. To effect a decisive shift we would have to have more sales staff, promotion, etc. All this would run into money and we have no guarantee that it actually would work. It may even backfire.'

It appeared that some manufacturers and, among them, one of the more important leaders in the industry, trade largely through wholesalers, and employ few salesmen. Non-leader executives declared that this pattern of distribution made them feel rather anxious when viewing the future. One of the men stated that wholesale distribution

'is not a pattern which a manufacturer of these household products starting today would adopt looking to the future. The fortunes of manufacturers who rely upon the wholesale trade for distributing their products are insecure. It depends whether in the future there will be an adequate margin of discount for the wholesaler, and this is uncertain in an age of growing opportunities in this business.'

Nevertheless, significantly, executives of this company saw their market as with the wholesaler and not with the consumer. One, in particular, was uncomfortable about the emphasis on wholesalers, a feeling which was aggravated by the fact that his company's sales directly to retailers and other outlets caused a certain amount of competitive friction. He defended himself against this anxiety by rationalizing the efforts designed to bring about a more evenly distributed sales set-up, with emphasis on retail outlets, as possibly too costly, i.e. 'it may not even work'.

The multiples, engaged in bulk-buying, appear to overshadow the smaller dealers in importance. Executives expressed themselves strongly in favour of rigorously structured trade discounts. They threatened and wished for penalties for violators. Referring to one competitor, suspected of disregarding strict trade discounts, one executive burst out: 'The business method of X [competitor] is a disgrace for [the country's] business. He should be driven out.'

But it was found that some of the very same executives, among them heads of divisions of world-renowned companies, did not in fact live up to their self-proclaimed standards. One of these men openly admitted that he had allowed an extra 15 per cent discount to a well-known multiple, and explained his action by saying that his factory had been running below capacity at the time.

Another interview produced the following:

'At whom do we aim our marketing efforts? You mean the selection of our customers? We try to avoid unequal distribution, the kind of competition which is unhealthy and not good for the industry. We are active, that is, I myself am very much interested in resale price maintenance. We believe in it. It is good and necessary for the industry, the dealers, and even for the protection of the consumer.'

The smaller household product dealers are generally not well thought of by these men. Both executives and staff of one non-leader company in particular often termed the operators of these outlets 'the lowest form of life'. It may be interesting to note that in the case of two household product groups, termed B and C in *Table 1*, which in recent years have found wider acceptance with the buying public, only a few companies still deal with wholesalers extensively. The majority now largely rely upon the retail outlets for their distribution. The companies who have done this most extensively are in the leader group.

(b) The Companies' Activities

(i) *Forward planning*. There was fairly general agreement among non-leader executives that little good could come by trying to plan in detail the company's activities in advance. One executive said:

'How do we determine the size of our production? We usually look at our figures of the previous years and if we think that prospects are good we add five per cent or so to last year's figures. Now sometimes this may not work too well. In 195X we could have sold many more of [product C] if we would have had them. Of course, there is no safe way in which one could predict demand. It depends on so many unknown factors. By comparison, you take [capital goods].'

A lengthy description of the advantages in planning production for these capital goods was then given.

Uncertainty about governmental policies in regard to credit, sales-tax, and instalment purchase regulations provides non-leader executives with another reason to devalue business programming. One said:

'You never know what they [the government] are going to do next. [In] 195X credit restrictions were removed and these household products sold well. The following year they were slapped right back again. And there you are. Would it have been wise to invest and expand your business?'

Discussing market research, the sales director of a non-leader company remarked that

'I know that American firms engage in large scale studies to find out all kinds of things. We believe that a lot of this is nonsense. One gets so much information that it becomes difficult to sift out what is important and what is not. Besides, who really understands women? We make household products which are serviceable, useful, they are well engineered, as well as or better than anyone else's. We price them so as to make a modest profit. It is really only a modest profit. Of course, it is the retailer's job to sell them directly to the consumer. He is equipped to do so. This is his function and he has his margin for this service.

38

Of course, we are guided by the principle to make the lot of the housewife easier. We want to help her. And, believe me, she has it a lot easier than when I was a boy.'

Another non-leader company participating in this study had an efficient and potentially very productive market research department. However, there was a paradoxical situation when it came to the use of this department. The divisions of this company that worked most efficiently availed themselves most of the facilities of the research department. Others, to whom a more intimate knowledge of their market would be of great value, used this type of research only marginally or not at all. This state of affairs was greatly defended as being inevitable with a limited budget. It turned out that the research budget of the company was divided among its divisions in accordance with their previous year's performance and not in accordance with their needs.

This arrangement savoured of circularity. It is like a man who is in poor condition because he does not have a balanced diet. In consequence his work suffers and his income decreases. To make ends meet he reduces his diet, which further reduces his efficiency, and so on.

Some executives rely upon members of their families and their friends for market information. The managing director of a household product division said:

'How do we get our information about what the consumer wants? Now, you take my daughter. She is married and has children. Whenever we go to her house for dinner I watch her. She is young, she is modern, she has ideas. I talk to her, I talk to her friends, they have plenty of new ideas. And, believe me, I have benefited from their advice and often it was quite critical. Then, also my door here is always open. Any of my men can come in here, and they

39

do. And they tell me things. And then we have our designing department; we send them out every two years to go to your country, America, and look round. We know. But . . . we are tied hand and foot by the dealers. They are the ones who really dictate to us.'

Other companies employ market researchers, either with independent agencies or in their own market research departments. It was rather surprising to note how often executives with non-leader firms equated and interchanged the terms 'market research' and 'marketing'.[1] One market researcher expressed himself with great emotion:

'My sales director is a ****. I bet in all the years since he left school, he had not read a half dozen books and they most likely were whodunits. He says: "Maybe next year we will be able to sell more . . . [household product]. What will the general economic conditions in the country be? Will they favour our sales campaign? Get me a picture of the *marketing* situation and a forecast." You see, he does not even know the meaning of the words *marketing* and *market research*. How can I tell him anything? He does not want to know why we don't sell. This is the death-wish. He wants excuses why we won't sell. When I try to tell him, he always says: "I know, I know". Does he know? How can I wake him up?'

The market researchers are rarely, if ever, asked to find out what is wrong or to work out recommendations how to improve conditions. Several reports shown to the author related to 'the inability of the Sales Department to perform

[1] *Market research* has been defined by the United States Department of Commerce as: 'The study of all problems relating to the transfer and sale of goods and services between producer and consumer . . . their physical distribution, wholesale and retail merchandising and financial problems concerned' (Market Research Agencies, 1932).

its function properly', i.e. to sell. These reports also referred to 'lack of co-ordination between Production, Advertising, and Sales Departments,' i.e. inadequate planning, at times placing the blame here and there, although carefully observing an indirect manner of expression. The author does not claim to have seen a large proportion of market research reports of non-leader firms. In fact, their actual number was eight, belonging to three companies. But the description given here is based on a carefully studied assessment. At no time has he seen with these firms a research report which analysed the position of a company and explained how this had come about. At no time did he see recommendations about what needed to be done expressed in a firm and clear manner and substantiated by evidence gained in the field.

Not a single marketing head sits on non-leader executive boards or boards of directors, i.e. has top-level management status. Their knowledge of top level business policy, wherever that clearly exists, is rather indirect. It is 'because the chairman' or 'a director let me know' and more often because 'knowing my people and analysing the questions they ask, what else can the policy be?' This surmise may often be quite correct. But it equally signifies that the marketing man is in no position to affect the situation one way or the other.

It has been found with these companies that size of production is often determined by executives who are removed from Sales and Marketing Departments where these exist. The sales directors were often found to be too timid to assert themselves and equally anxious to disengage themselves from responsibility. In these instances the profits of the household product divisions, in so far as the information was made available to the author, were limited. At times there were even losses. In two companies the policy of keeping the household product division going was largely based on a desire 'not to lose face in the industry'.

41

(ii) *Product planning.* Three factors became discernible with non-leader companies whose executives openly admitted that their household product division operated 'far less successfully than desired'. These companies had a widely diversified range of household products. There was an appreciable lack of cost-consciousness. They insisted on a *perfect* product and not a *marketable* product.

Some executives stated that they 'must offer the distributors and dealers a wide range of products'. Directly linked to this consideration, decisions with respect to the use of resources were not always determined by expected profitability. In at least one instance, in an account of how a decision was reached, neither product nor market was stressed. Treating both rather lightly, it was the head of the division, 'John, who got the money and production. He is the kind of chap you just can't say no to.'

Demonstrating lack of cost-consciousness and insistence on a *perfect* product one chief executive of a non-leader firm said:

'We have this—[household product] model. It is a first class—[household product]. When the mock-up came from Designing, some of us in Production looked it over. It looked all right but technically we had to make some changes. After all, we have an obligation to our high standard of reputation. And then Sales comes around and tells us that our changes substantially increased the retail price which makes it difficult to sell the item. Hell! The changes were worth far more. We are not going to cheapen ourselves. What's more, our price was in line with most of our competitors.'

Another executive said:

'Styling? Now you know we are entirely dependent on the dealers. For instance, there would be no point in making

42

products with perfect consumer satisfaction. We must get acceptance from the dealers. Ease of service, deliveries, trade discounts, that is what they are looking for. Although we know what is right for the consumer, we must accept the dictates of the dealers, prejudiced as they may be.'

But this was not the only instance when executives tried to impress on the author that their efforts on product-planning were decisively guided by the whims of dealers. Another executive, relying on the counsels of his wife, seemed to place the desires of the market into a rather obscure position. He said:

'On designing, my wife is a first-class designer. She does it all by herself, though I help her a bit. We always have the sketches checked by a panel of experts and they give us a 1A. But last year we sent them out for a public test. The results of this test were not in line with the results of the panel. And now my wife won't do it any more. How do you explain this? . . . Well, it is really simple. It just proves how far ahead we are of them.'

It appears that household products of non-leaders are well made. They are designed by engineers. But stylists and marketing people have little say in this matter.

(iii) *Advertising*. Judging by the market shares, the advertising policies of the non-leader companies cannot be held to be particularly successful. Interviews with executives of these firms indicated a surprising belief in what advertising can do. One, for example, asserted that 'a company image can be created according to a design, almost *in vacuo*'. This image, another believed, 'can be shaped in accordance with what a company *needs to be* so as to make a desired impression, and this irrespective of what the company actually might *happen to be*'.

43

This last quoted expression came after a protracted interview in the course of which the executive, holding the rank of a deputy chairman in his company, displayed great anxiety about the market position of his firm's household product division and developed his ideas on how he intended it to 'Americanize' and to 'streamline'.

Some executives considered snob-appeal of prime importance in advertising. In response to probing the attitudes towards socio-economic groups, executives declared, at times with great emotion, that they were correct to slant their promotion towards the upper and upper-middle classes. These groups, of course, are also those which executives themselves belong to but do not necessarily come from. Some executives asserted that 'the working-classes are positively affected by snob-appeal, i.e. they like to identify themselves with the upper classes.' This again may well have expressed a projection of this group's own feelings. There were no research data available to corroborate this belief.

Another non-leader company felt the need to effect a change in its advertising approach and seriously considered removing its account to another agency. During the period of uncertainty no less than seven different tentative campaigns were planned for it. Finally the account was left with the original agency. But instead of changing the advertising approach, it was decided to change the account executive. More than a year later, there was still no significant change in the company's advertising approach or its sales figures. But the sales figures for the industry as a whole had risen.

At this stage it seemed worth while to make some investigation of the creative method of the agency concerned. The author arranged for five individual meetings and one group meeting with members of the agency. They involved the organization's account director, the account manager, the 'economic' researcher, the creative executive, and the

44

copy executive, all concerned with the non-leader firm's advertisements. The attitudes about methods employed in the development of advertisements that emerged from these meetings indicate a close similarity between the frame of mind and the views of the agency's executives and those in the company. In the course of the interviews it became clear that the agency, like the company it worked for, had little faith in the value of consumer research. The company's advertisements were not systematically pre-tested, and when consumer research was carried out it was liable to be sent to America to be evaluated. Executives of the company were aware of this but seemed unworried. They were then asked whether it would be satisfactory for their products to be designed at a place several thousand miles away. There was no answer. The agency prided itself on 'penetrating the minds of the public' in the same way that the company executives were sure that they knew what the public wanted and what it ought to have.

As representative of a cross-section of these executives' views on advertising, the following can be cited: 'Promotion? You mean advertising? Well, of course, we must go on advertising. We must keep our name in front of the public. But how much does it help sales?'

(iv) *Selling*. Top-level executives of all companies when interviewed expressed their concern about adequate sales incentives. When developing such a system they experienced considerable difficulties. Some of these difficulties were real and objective. Others were not explicable in terms of business. One was the concept that the company's representatives, as gentlemen, were trusted to do their best. The introduction of sales targets and commissions would make them feel distrusted, would cause petty rivalries among them, and thus eventually prove disadvantageous to the company's operation.

It was worth noting that the predominant attitude permeating this sales force was that the relation between salesman and buyer could be seen as a social call between gentlemen. This was highlighted by the reply of the sales manager of this non-leader firm to a question by the author about the number of calls his salesmen were expected to make on their accounts and how this was supervised. 'Sir', he answered, 'the calls of a salesman on his accounts are a personal matter between him and his account. I would never interfere there.'

Additional expressions of attitudes towards selling were found in some of the 'send-offs' salesmen received from their superiors when launching a new product. From a number of sales meetings attended by the author the following excerpts may best demonstrate this.

'I shall now unveil to you the latest models in—[product] our engineers have produced. The brand name [blank] has been chosen wisely. There is nothing finer in the market either with our competitors or elsewhere in this world. Now here—(description of features, colours, variations between a *de luxe* and a *super de luxe* brand). We shall be able to make our first impact on the market in— [month] backed up by deliveries first with smaller quantities, but then with increasing momentum.'

'Now I know you would like better deliveries and so would I. But ours is not to reason why. We must act. We must sell. This occasion reminds me so strongly of when during the last war our troops received—[a type of artillery]. It may not have been the turning-point of the war, but . . ..'

The basic attitude seemed to be that in which the decision about the product was made first. When presenting the product to the salesmen this attitude remained predominant.

46

It was not specifically related to the market. Comments of salesmen attending the meeting indicated that the brand name of the products might sound impressive, but the brands themselves were not much, if at all, different from those of competitors.

The reverse side of the coin is seen when production men or top-level managers consider the request of Sales for innovations, i.e. product advantages, merely as frills and consequently as quite unnecessary.

(c) Attitudes towards Household Products

Executives of non-leaders in the industry – among them the larger companies – seemed to have a particular attitude towards household products. Time and again they expressed sentiments according to which dealing with household products represented a quasi apprenticeship or trial period. 'Once', some commented, 'they have shown their mettle', i.e. made good in this department, they will be promoted to medium and large products, the stuff that 'really counted'. Moreover, promotion to the board of such a company was considered likely from the latter two divisions only. To move up from the household product division directly seemed exceptional.

This attitude was displayed more dramatically by one executive when comparing the advantages of planning the production of capital goods as opposed to household products (see page 38). He went on: 'Now by comparison take this [household product].' He extended his left arm to pick up a household product from his desk. Although it was within comfortable reach of his hand, he used his nails and finger tips to bring it closer to himself. After explaining several improvements of it, he put it back in its original place on the desk, always handling it with fingertips and nails.

'You see how many advantages it has. From a production engineer's point of view it is as good as can be made for the market. But do housewives buy it as they should? They really don't know what they want.'

With this he took a handkerchief from his breastpocket and wiped his fingers.

The shift in the interview from the discussion about capital goods to the household product was dramatically underlined by a change in the executive's behaviour. From a slouching position gradually developed during the course of the conversation, when the subject related to household products only, he suddenly and almost instantaneously sat up straight when mentioning industrial products and capital goods. His whole manner changed and became firmer. A high pitch changed into a well-modulated, sonorous tone of voice. The subject of industrial products, not directly related to the purpose of the interview, occupied a considerable period of time. This obviously was a field of business which a man like him could enjoy. It seemed to have an aspect of glamour and masculine construction. Against this, the handling and description of the household product were marked by a sharp contrast. Here the executive played two roles. One, the engineer who had made a wonderful product, technically unassailable. In the other, the researcher gained the impression that this executive felt himself nagged by the housewife, who failed to appreciate just anything. The household product itself, handled with fingertips and nails, must have been felt as quite uncomfortable, a feeling which necessitated the wiping of his fingers with the handkerchief. A subsequent inspection by the author showed the household product to be immaculately clean.

Increasingly an impression conveyed itself that to the non-leader executives the ultimate consumer and even their own products, while supplying the basis of their livelihood, are nevertheless both feared and disliked. As a result, their dependence on both consumer and products appears more in the form of hanging on to something that is hated rather than serving someone who is felt to be good.

(d) The Consumer

In the course of interviews with non-leader executives, the researcher probed their concepts of consumer-housewives. It appeared characteristic of these men to stress to a magnified degree and, at times at least, out of sequence, their 'concern for women', their 'desire to serve women', 'to improve their lot'. This was interspersed with complaints about the 'difficulty of understanding women', expressed, at least at one level, as chagrin about 'female inability to make rational purchase decisions'. Invariably, however, such complaints were followed by assurances that the executive harboured 'no prejudice against women'. One stated: 'The ultimate consumer? You mean the housewife? Well, I must admit, we really do not know as much about her as we should. You could say that we really do not know her at all.'

This, however, was patently untrue. His company had employed for several years a number of women demonstrators, most of whom were housewives, all of whom sold the company's products in retail outlets to housewives. Information which the company extracted from their experience was about the housewife. Furthermore, with the considerable amount of social research done in the country concerned, both academically and commercially, a great deal of revelant information is available. The executive's assertion that 'we really do not know her at all' is symptomatic of his anxiety about the amount of knowledge of the housewife he permits himself to have. He might have more correctly stated

49

his feeling by saying: '. . . we really do not know as much about her as our business would require'.

More illuminating was an interview with another member of the same firm. He said:

'Now, I am glad that you ask me about the users of our household products. There was a time when we sold to the better middle classes. You know, the backbone of the country. These days we have a new orientation. We practically sell to anyone who has the money to buy. Now this is a fine thing. But do you know who buys our products? My gardener does! And I must tell you about him. His two children, a boy and a girl, went to college just like my son did. They are both working, having fine jobs. He is working and his wife is working. And what do they do with their money? I tell you! The other day I had occasion to drive by his house and visit him. Don't ask me why! Do you know what they buy? A stupid television set. Here we spend thousands on medical research to show how important it is for the health of people to buy our [household products]. But do they take advantage of it? I still think that we should make an exclusive line for the businessman, the professional man, the middle-class white-collar man. We would avoid much trouble.'

It was noticeable that this executive criticized the working classes for buying TV sets and not his firm's household products. He expressed indignation that they should thereby implicitly criticize his own efforts at giving them what he thought was best for them. He further implied that nowadays working class people are far too well off for their own good.

On four occasions, a preoccupation with the Near East market was discernible. This, considering the political and economic conditions prevailing there, was rather strange.

50

Alerted by the repeating pattern, the researcher was able in the course of one interview to note the following answer to the question: 'To whom do you sell your products?'

A detailed, non-technical description of a sale to a Near East royal palace was given. It lasted for twenty-two minutes of the interview. The job amounted to the equivalent of $5,500.

It was followed by a description of a major industrial job abroad. It lasted for five minutes of the interview. The job amounted to the equivalent of $13.5 million.

After a few seconds of silence, the answer to this question was completed by this sentence: 'And there is, of course, the general public.' These sales to the general public totalled a multiple of the aforementioned figure of $13.5 million.

This executive's interest, at least on a manifest level, was not centred on the general public in his own country, which absorbed the bulk of his company's production, but rather on smaller and obviously to him more glamorous sectors of the company's business. Yet his concern for the type of overseas business he talked about should not be mistaken for a preoccupation with exports. This he brought out clearly in the course of conversation. The obvious relish with which he described the royal household made it clear that it was the glamour of the assignment rather than its contribution to exports which appealed to him.

In a subsequent joint interview, another executive, in charge of the marketing policy of the same company, argued similarly against using a type of sales promotion with which consumers in the working classes could readily identify themselves. He thought that to encourage workers to acquire possessions which so far they had not enjoyed would provide further incentive for higher wage demands, and 'add more stimuli to inflation'. Moreover, he continued, 'expansion of domestic sales will result in lower export sales and higher import prices. The expenditure on household consumer goods has increased too much already.' His colleague, previously interviewed, expressed full agreement with his point of view.

Executives, particularly among non-leaders, often admitted that their sales promotion is narrowly directed to the middle and upper classes. This group of consumers, however, is limited:

1. in its numbers (less than 25 per cent of the total population),
2. in its spending pattern, since so much of its income goes on education, housing, and holidays.

(e) Government Policies and Regulations

It has been pointed out before that some non-leader executives thought programming their companies' business activities to be of little avail because repeated changes in governmental regulations and policies made this impossible (see page 38). Another executive said:

'The government is responsible for making prices grossly inflated (by levying sales taxes on [household products]) and thereby deters the public from buying these products.'

A frequently mentioned subject was resale price maintenance. To quote one executive:

'Resale price maintenance avoids destructive price and profit warfare, destructive to the dealers and the industry as a whole. It prevents the bad elements in business from coming to the top, those who fake and cheat, who do not give value, the foreign element on the [national] scene. But more than that, it brings out the best in dealers, better sales personnel, better service personnel.'

(f) The Successful Competitor

One recurring feature is the feeling expressed about success-ful competitors, a feeling that appears to be a compound of puzzlement and resentment. The following comment is characteristic of this:

'Now our competitors. You know, I refer to those who are called specialists. They make only a few household products, they specialize in them. Now we make an— [household product] which is as good as theirs and better. We would not stoop to some of their tricks. But they cater to the women. Now we have to do the same. We have demonstrators out in the field just as they do. The fact is, we have everything they have got. But they are the specialists, and all these women run to buy their stuff.'

On the surface it is very difficult to know what to make of these remarks. 'Catering to women' appears equated with 'tricks' to which the company of this executive 'would not stoop'. However, some form of 'catering' seems acceptable and is even imitated. Later, it even seems that the imitation is viewed as complete, i.e. 'the fact is, we have everything they have got'. Yet, women seem to prefer the 'specialists' stuff', which obviously baffles the executive. The explanation would seem to be the strong feeling expressed by this execu-tive about women and their whims, shown for example in the derogatory term he used in the phrase 'all these women'. These comments contain fear of and contempt for the house-wife, and it is difficult to believe that these feelings could not interfere with successful selling. The imitation may be far-reaching, but the admixture of fear and contempt tends to distort details of the 'catering' effect sufficiently to cancel substantial portions of its intended effect.

There was also great intensity of feeling against successful competitors, particularly those who can be branded as 'outsiders'. The sales manager of another company exclaimed:

'Look who is successful in selling household products in this country. Americans, Jews, Quakers. You don't find an honest to goodness [national] in the whole blooming lot.'

In fact, there is an amazingly inconsistent pattern. It is, by and large, the 'outsiders' who have brought innovation in marketing, production, and even financial and administrative techniques to the industry. If there is insufficient innovation and insufficient production on the part of the native producers, it is not surprising that 'outsiders' should have such a large measure of success. It is possible, of course, that the depth of feeling can be explained as an emotional reaction to competition affecting one's livelihood. This would be equally irrational, however, since these successful competitors have in the course of their innovatory efforts expanded the whole market and thus indirectly benefited all manufacturers in the industry.

(g) General Attitudes and Aptitudes

Inevitably in highlighting particular topics, for which the non-leader executives' attitudes can be regarded as significant, their viewpoints and responses in what might be described as 'non-sensitive' areas are omitted. Thus, it is possible that a ludicrously one-sided and therefore misleading image of their personalities and capabilities may be given to the reader. It should, therefore, be emphasized that it is not suggested and it would not be justifiable to conclude that there is any general lack of ability among these men, here termed non-leader executives. Perhaps the most striking

54

single feature that this study brought out is that time and again these same executives gave proof of great ability when dealing with products other than household. The great majority of them had worked themselves up to their present positions of responsibility through other divisions of their companies. They had given proof time and again of their ability. However, in their other responsibilities they were almost invariably dealing, not with the general public and with housewives, particularly working-class housewives, but with large organizations, government departments, industrial undertakings, and other such bodies. The same executives who seem unable to market household products successfully have been able to organize the production of industrial equipment and can successfully market medium and large-sized products.

There is, of course, the point that for nearly twenty years, during World War II and during the period of post-war restriction, production was one of the industry's most important problems. The effort to maintain production in the face of shortages, labour difficulties, and government restrictions was accompanied by problems of finance created by the credit restrictions, and this at a time of constantly rising costs. To overcome it, the industry developed first-class production techniques and astute financial management. As a result, top-level executives, at least among non-leaders, usually came from engineering, finance, and production, and only in a few instances from sales or marketing.

There is a further point that a feature of many of the non-leader companies is a high degree of diversification; that is to say that household products are not the only or even the main part of their business, but one among a variety of products. The leaders in the industry are, in general, household product 'specialists'.

It might at first sight seem that these factors in themselves provide an explanation for the relative lack of success among non-leaders. The significant feature, however, is not that a large company manufacturing a wide variety of products should occasionally fail with one or other of them, but that it should invariably be household products that represent the unsuccessful effort. The significance of this is not lost on the executives themselves; many gave evidence of considerable anxiety on this score: the executive who complained about the lack of consumer acceptance for his product (see page 48), and another deploring women's preference for 'specialists' stuff' (see page 53). Many more who expressed themselves in the same sense bear this out.

There were further signs of anxiety in the form of self-questioning about the role of the executive, of their companies, and of business generally in the life of the community. Some held that 'the paramount purpose of business is profit'. This view was opposed by others who contended that: 'business must primarily provide a service to the community, considering profits almost as a by-product of its activities.' Many gave, at least at a superficial level, the impression that they were dedicated to the welfare of the housewife. They reiterated their 'concern for women', their 'desire to serve women', 'to improve their lot' (see page 49). One top-level executive got very heated in the course of the interview. He exclaimed:

> 'We rest on a great tradition. If one were to listen to some people, we are all through. I will not say that we are the cornerstone of our country if you like, but we are one of the most important industries and by God we are aware of our responsibilities.'

This was part of the response to the question: 'To whom do you sell your products?'

The following dialogue gives further evidence on this point.

EXECUTIVE: Do you think that a sales director should be the best salesman in the country, or should he be a leader of men?

AUTHOR: This is a very interesting problem. I never encountered it in such pure form. I would have to think about this. But, obviously, you must have given it much thought. I would be greatly interested to learn your opinion.

EXECUTIVE: I have never done much selling . . . I am a leader of men. I know what moves them, how they work, what will make them work. But the important part is to control your plant. If you have a plant, selling comes automatically. If you concentrate on sales only, you have nothing.

It should be explained that this company was one of those which had seriously considered disbanding its household product division because of its lack of success. Yet the dialogue presents an executive who is anxious about the role of salesmanship, aware of his company's failure in this respect, and yet insisting: 'If you have a plant, selling comes automatically.' This was a statement which his own experience had proved to be untrue.

It can be seen from this that there would be no justification for a charge of smugness against these men. There is a sincere effort to find remedies and a considerable amount of soul-searching, which, however, seemingly ends in helpless resignation.

It may be asked how general attitudes like these are throughout the non-leader companies. In the course of the study the opportunity was taken to examine the companies' policy-decision-making procedure. It was found that in most cases one man was responsible for the ultimate decisions. In no instance were there more than four individuals involved and where there was an apparent division of power invariably one individual carried greatest weight. The tone was set by the man at the top, although at least in two cases nominal and functional leaders were not identical. This tone penetrated the hierarchy with individuals in subordinate positions echoing these attitudes. It may be fruitless to examine whether they held their jobs because they shared the attitude of top management, or whether they shared the attitudes because they held the jobs. In either case there was an effective homogeneity.

PROFILE OF NON-LEADER SALESMEN

The other group profile which evolved from the material gathered in the course of the main pilot study was that of non-leader salesmen. Essentially its main features can be summarized as:

(*a*) attitudes towards the job, and
(*b*) attitudes towards consumers.

(*a*) Attitudes towards the Job

It appeared that the non-leader salesmen heavily relied upon buyers in the trade, i.e. wholesalers, retailers, multiples, etc., to do them a 'favour' as friends. The salesmen felt obliged 'to unload the company's products' and expected 'the buyer to buy'. They seemed to prefer the 'old boy' approach, and this regardless of the buyer's preference, which tended towards a sales story, preferably a 'unique selling point', i.e. product advantages.

Forty-three salesmen in three companies were presented with projective devices. One item in a sentence completion read: THE RELATIONSHIP BETWEEN BUYER AND SALESMAN— —————————————————————————. Thirty-one salesmen when completing this sentence used the terms 'friendship' or 'mutual aid'.

58

To three TAT-type sketches, relevant to this relationship (see Appendix A, items 1, 2, and 3), about two-thirds of the responses referred to buying new stocks. Only 28 responses out of a total of 129 (less than 22 per cent) used an expression like 'the salesman will sell'. Nearly all other responses were expressed in terms of 'the salesman will get an order' or 'the buyer will buy'.

Sales representatives of one non-leader company made at least one unsuccessful attempt to be called *salesmen* and not *travellers*. It is not particularly surprising that there was a great sensitivity on the score of their position and standing. It is understandable in the light of general business practice. The 'salesman' or 'representative' is generally held to have a higher social standing than a 'traveller'. The implication of the latter term is that he deals with a large number of products from different firms, while the former works directly for a single company. What was significant in this instance, however, was that the request for the higher status title, which would have cost nothing, was unhesitatingly refused.

It may not be coincidence that this company did not set sales targets either for its household products division or for the salesmen. Possibly a sufficiently high salary and a higher social status accorded to the job could have provided an adequate incentive to pursue a vigorous sales policy but, in the absence of these, the lack of sales targets meant that the salesmen had no incentive, negative or positive, to greater efforts. The only way in which they could hope to increase their incomes was by being promoted. This, however, represented a long-term goal so remote that it could not have much effect upon their day-to-day efforts. On the other hand, although the job offered little hope of advancement, it certainly appeared secure. These were ideal conditions for producing apathy.

However, even if the salesman was an ambitious, energetic individual he still could not afford to antagonize his colleagues by doing so much better than the average. Social pressure is often irresistible. Although he may feel guilty about doing less than his best, he would feel more guilty if he were to break the unwritten code as to what constitutes a fair day's work. As a result, these salesmen, although not very well paid, present, nevertheless, in reality a picture that mirrors fairly accurately the image of them held by non-leader executives.

(i) They are expensive to the company when measured by their results.

(ii) They, seemingly, enjoy security in their jobs.

Beneath this security, however, is a nagging doubt about their future should the household product division of their company be dissolved because of unsatisfactory business results, i.e. lack of profits. This is not an unrealistic fear. Two of the companies among the non-leader group had at one time or other seriously considered disbanding their household product division. They had been deterred from doing so, apparently only in the last analysis, by the fear of loss of prestige.

That this apathy was a matter of lack of incentive rather than a lack of sales ability was made clear on the odd occasion when a cash incentive had been introduced. When merchandise did not move for some time, one of the companies in the non-leader group offered a commission on the sale of it. It then moved. By withholding the opportunity of increased income due to stepped-up sales, by paying commissions on slow-moving items, often at reduced prices, policy-making executives in essence placed a premium on sales lethargy. In a sense the salesmen had a negative incentive to sell the company's products. It was only when a product was slow to move that they were paid extra to sell it.

Two other companies had a sales target system. However, both salesmen and executives below the policy-making level termed it 'unrealistic'.

It also deserves consideration that nearly all these salesmen, while trying to maintain a middle-class standard, whatever that may have meant to them, earned less than the equivalent of $2,500 per annum. This made it difficult for them to buy for their own use the products which it was their job to sell.

(b) *Attitudes towards Consumers*

Some interviews with members of this group of salesmen produced strong expressions of resentment against the 'now prosperous working classes'. When presenting three additional TAT-type sketches, depicting kitchens stocked with household products in varying numbers, the respondents were asked to describe the people who lived in these houses, their ages, occupations, and characters.

In response to a drawing of a kitchen heavily stocked with household products, the average profile was:

Husband about 33 years old, professional man or executive, upper income bracket, the equivalent of about $5,500 annual income. Wife about 29 years old. Two small children. The family was pictured as easy-going, tidy, intellectual, broad-minded, and liking entertainment.

The response profile to the drawing showing a kitchen minimally stocked with household products was:

Husband about 55 years old, manual labourer, annual income the equivalent of about $1,800. Wife about 50 years old. Two or three children, either having left home or going to work. The family was pictured as untidy, old-fashioned, unintelligent, stupid, devoid of character.

The response profile to a drawing showing a kitchen averagely stocked with household products was:

Husband about 35 years old, clerk or factory worker. Wife about 32 years old, a part-time worker. Two children in the family. The family was pictured as tidy but struggling, in trouble, as a result of having 'modern or American ideas'.

The drawings were all identical, except for the number of household products drawn on each. Consequently either all or none could have produced a perception of being tidy or untidy, at times expressed in terms of 'dirty' and 'stinking'.

Responses to the projective devices confirmed the impressions gained in interviews and while accompanying these salesmen on their calls on customers. Rarely did references to the housewife-consumer suggest that she was thought of as a complete person, really liked and understood. Members of the 'now prosperous working classes' were portrayed as 'socially beneath the level of the salesmen themselves'. The fact that nowadays this group of consumers can afford to purchase these household products was often brought forth in a tone of voice or with accompanying gestures that indicated envy. This envy found more concrete expression when these salesmen discussed with retail floor-salesmen points in favour of their products. Invariably these salesmen's points were of a technical nature, difficult to understand for the average housewife and consequently not of great interest to her. Obviously, they fell short of being a convincing sales argument.

On several occasions, and in the presence of the author, retail salesmen conveyed this to the non-leader representatives, while pointing to advertisements and other promotional material of leaders which they believed to contain a 'good sales story'. The non-leader salesmen's answer that they carried out instructions received at their offices was most likely correct but of little relevance. Since these were not isolated complaints the question arises why the salesmen failed to change their approach, whether backed by their offices or not.

THE PSYCHOLOGY OF THE NON-LEADERS

Both the successful companies and the non-leaders provided the author with a wealth of material, but one significant difference must be emphasized. Alexander and his team provided and were ready to permit the use of a great deal of material related to their personal backgrounds. In addition, these men made no reference to and had no complaints about changing social conditions in the country. By contrast the non-leader executives were much less ready to permit the use of personal material and seemed in many instances to be deeply concerned with the social conditions surrounding them. Both the successful and the non-leader companies were facing the same social and general environmental conditions. Certain psychological inferences are strongly suggested by this. The non-leader executives appear to have personal conflicts directly affecting their business which are not resolved. They deal with these conflicts by displacing them into the social sphere. The successful companies' executives seem to have been able to resolve these personal problems within the context of their business. They have, therefore, apparently no need for such displacement. The following is concerned with presenting the evidence leading to this conclusion.

There have been various attempts in the past to explain business success or the lack of it. Some have attempted to relate it to the innate capability of the executives concerned: to say, in other words, that the good ones are successful and the bad ones are not. This, however, explains nothing. It merely repeats the basic situation with the addition of two emotive words. A slightly deeper analysis is found in the suggestion that it takes managements a period of time to adjust themselves to changing social and economic conditions and that some adjust themselves quicker than others. Adler (1956), for example, argues that managements steeped in past social and economic patterns are taking a long time to incorporate the changes that have taken place in purchasing power into their thinking. The new customers are obviously there and the managements are prepared to pay lip-service to their existence. But they do not act as though they believed in their existence. Although this theory is a step along the road it raises more questions than it explains. Why, for example, does one management have no difficulty in accepting the facts of the social situation while another finds this almost impossible?

It might be argued that management in viewing its markets suffers from its conventional business experience and training in economics. This, it is asserted, may be an example of Bartlett's (1932) proposed pattern thinking, in which it is assumed that characteristics of institutions and mechanisms are stressed in preference to people and their wants. Hence the acceptance of reality is delayed.

It might be assumed that these executives cannot believe the evidence before their eyes, because they do not want to believe it. Such executives appear to be emotionally denying the practical existence of facts, although simultaneously the existence of these facts is intellectually admitted; these executives may be said to be engaged in an unconscious denial of business reality. Psycho-analytic theory informs us that the denial of reality may represent an unconscious

64

defence against unbearable anxiety. Two questions then arise:

(i) How does the defence operate in this instance? and
(ii) What is the nature of the anxiety?

As a result of contact with non-leader executives, evidence with an essentially cumulative impact has been collected. It conveyed the impression that these executives tried to diminish contact with household products by viewing them in a deprecating manner, particularly when compared to industrial products and capital goods. This attitude, however, often broke down with the awareness, conscious and unconscious, that it diminishes the value both of the household products and, in turn, of the executives themselves to their own companies. This, then, caused another defence, displacing this deprecating attitude from the product on to the housewife-consumer, the user of the products.

It has been pointed out that household products in the country today have two functions. Overtly, their purpose is to aid the housewife in her chores. However, in making life easier for her, household products acquire another, although more latent, function: they represent symbols of social and economic well-being (see pages 29–30). As such they were once widely considered the prerogative of the country's upper and middle classes, not generally available to the working classes. Moreover, the use of the working class as servants with long hours at work may also have served the function of immobilizing them as potentially dangerous upsetters of the social order – a fear that can today be seen in the 'colour problem' countries.

It would appear that among companies successful in the industry the attitudes of their executives are marked by a desire to manufacture and sell their household products, limited only by conditions of business reality. Among the non-leader companies these attitudes of executives seem to be of an ambivalent character. At a conscious level they obviously wish to fulfil their business function, that is, to sell the products of their companies to potential customers. Yet, in the actual marketing performance, there appears a resistance. This resistance is related to the two functions of the products mentioned before. It is of a complex and largely unconscious nature; it tends to cancel some of the consciously exerted sales efforts.

The desire to resist social change finds expression in a 'split' image of consumers. An analysis of the material evolved from the pilot study indicated that many of these executives had an image of consumer-housewives which can be termed 'split' in the clinical sense. One part was influenced by the perception of their wives and of friends in their own social class. Another part presented itself with features of a working class which had progressed 'beyond its station'. It contained such unflattering and stereotyped features as being irresponsible (gambling on pools, dog races, etc.), docile, and childish (addiction to TV and other spectator activities), unmindful of their health (rejection of hygiene by failing to acquire products C), irrational and profligate (impulse buying of useless trifles instead of household products).

This picture demonstrates a striking similarity with the one held by salesmen of these companies (see pages 58–63). It provides evidence for the observation that the entire hierarchy of a company tends to identify with the attitudes held by its executives, a phenomenon first noted by Freud, in his *Group Psychology and the Analysis of the Ego* (1922).

The unflattering picture of the working-class housewife serves a manifold purpose. It reduces the number of potential consumers for household products in the minds and consequently the marketing plans of these executives. It neatly categorizes the 'difficult group' within a widely accepted classification – the working classes. It can then be readily believed that it is this broad group of the population which has *separated itself* from the benefits which the makers of household products could bestow upon them. It camouflages the executives' resentment against the 'now prosperous' working classes which achieve 'consumer comfort by rising incomes . . . and are unfairly luckier than [the executives themselves] were as boys – [and thereby] are getting above their stations'.

By way of compensation, the rest of the consumer population, the middle and upper classes, become more important, and a promotional and sales approach largely directed towards them becomes justified. It beguiles these executives into the belief that they have no prejudice against women *per se*. It also helps to reinforce other cherished prejudices of a social nature. Mainly, however, it demonstrates that broad groups of the population cannot be counted among prospects and, even if they were, they would be really incapable of appreciating true value. This, then, places the onus for the low market shares of the companies on these groups of consumers whose capabilities are inadequate for the job; the fault lies in a huge sector of the consumer potential which fails to play its part in the national economy correctly. And, indeed, those executives are not incompetent at all; this they successfully prove when dealing with the 'big stuff' and the 'big customers' such as governments or organizations as massive as their own.

It has already been suggested that the discussion of the problem in social terms is a reflection or displacement of the deeper psychological situation. The question now arises of what essentially this situation is. One clue to this problem is provided by the attitude of the non-leader executives towards consumer-housewives. It has been shown earlier in the text (see pages 49–54) that, in spite of the frequent expressions of 'concern for women' and a desire 'to improve their lot', there were complaints of difficulty in understanding women and female irrationality. Moreover, working-class housewives were in general felt to be irresponsible and childish, and their spending habits were roundly condemned.

Another clue can be found in the readiness of these executives to belittle household products, a subject which has also been dealt with above. This attitude, at a deeper level, correlated handling household products with being of a female or incomplete male status, i.e. young adolescent-like status. Household products are essentially made and sold to aid women in their household chores—washing, cleaning, handling of food. These are by tradition female activities, associated with the image of the good mother. This places some executives in a situation of conflict. The job of marketing these products effectively requires identification with the female role or 'the need to put oneself in the housewife's shoes'. Medium and heavy industrial products and the capital goods of the industry represent in this culture symbols of male functions. To market these is more glamorous and masculine. Consequently, to move up from household products to medium and heavy industrial equipment represents to these executives, albeit mostly at an unconscious level, the process of being initiated into full manhood. To remain, in turn, at the low-status household product level seems to stand for being unworthy of promotion to full manhood, and being judged to be good only to deal at a female level.

It should be noted, however, that apparently among the successful companies, the other leaders as they emerged from the material collected in the course of this study, this attitude does not seem to prevail. There the ambitious executive can show his best only with household goods,

These companies or groups of companies usually do not manufacture anything else. It may be that this lack of variation in products makes it easier for these men to identify with female functions in the use of these products. Moreover, it appears that executives who for this and other even deeper-lying personal motives manifest resistance to effective attitudes in marketing household products simply leave the leader companies. It has also been mentioned that a considerable amount of material displaying personal conflicts in non-leader executives and affecting their business functions, although at an unconscious level, has been eliminated from this study at the request of these executives. It should be said, however, that no single predominant syndrome or pattern of early environmental background could be detected or is claimed for this group of executives.

But there is one suggestive piece of evidence that should be mentioned at this time. While collecting the material, the author was struck by the fact that four executives in two separate companies, in reply to the question: 'To whom do you sell your products?', made particular and emphatic mention of the royal families of the Near East. As remarked earlier in the text, this emphasis seemed odd in view of the political and economic conditions prevailing in this area and also of its objective insignificance as a market for the companies' products. Why should it loom so large? This can be interpreted on at least two levels. The obvious theme is snobbery, with a deeper connotation that these executives are dissociating themselves as far as possible from the working-class market and heading as far above it as it is possible to do. Moreover, by implication at least, this emphasis tends to devalue the role of household products themselves. If one's chief pride is selling them to absolute monarchs who are surrounded by every sort of servant, then the household product itself can hardly be regarded as particularly essential. It is almost as though the executives were saying: 'Who buys our goods? People who do not need them!'

Second, there is beneath these words just a suggestion that it is a royal family that buys their products and accepts their worth, and thus it is there that the executives are most at home and not among the broad general public in the country whom they really do not like and who, they feel, do not like them or their products. This implies a fantasy of really being a prince, a member of a royal family, destined for the 'higher things in life'. But being placed in the present, non-royal environment by misfortune, one is separated from one's own 'good mother' by a witch, a 'bad mother', and forced to busy oneself with the 'lower things in life'.

The question must now be asked: 'Why was it necessary, at least for a number of non-leader executives, to stress repeatedly that they 'have no prejudice against women?' The answer to this question points to the character structure of executives containing unresolved anxieties about their own masculinity. They suffer doubts, largely unconscious, about the adequacy with which they fulfil their roles as husbands, fathers, and heads of households. Dealing with these household products, and the need for identification with the female role in the use of them, makes it seem to these men that when acting out a female role they become less masculine. This intensifies their anxiety. To diminish it defences mentioned before are invoked.

This syndrome of attitudes resulted, at least with one company, in a sales approach in which two factors were predominant. One could best be described as a cold-blooded wooing of the housewife. It was designed to move cold-bloodedly household products from the company's plants into the homes of the consumer, and cash from the consumer's paypacket into the cash register of the company. The cloven hoof of this wooing, as indeed of any cold-blooded wooing, was inevitably contempt for the wooed, although cloaked in paternalistic benevolence.

The other side of the coin depicted the housewife as a purchasing agent who carefully considers economic and functional factors and then consciously proceeds to consummate well thought-out buying decisions. Both these approaches were quite manifest in the sales, promotion, advertising and service of the company. They had two factors in common:

(i) They were barren of any real warmth towards the consumer.

(ii) They had not produced results to the satisfaction of the company.

V. Universal

Universal, as has been pointed out earlier, is a division of a firm in this household product industry which has moved from among the group of non-leaders to that of the leaders, and this in a relatively short period of time. Among the non-leaders described, managements remained unchanged in personnel and also appeared homogeneous among themselves in character and attitudes at least as far as they are related to business. At Universal there had been a recent change of top-level management. It became apparent that the present and previous management teams differed widely not only in their performances but also in their attitudes towards business. Since reference to this condition comes out throughout the material presented here, it will be useful to give an account of the history of this change in development.

Originally Universal made only industrial products and none for household use. In the 1920s one of its divisions started to make a limited number of household products, but its new off-shoot operated only on a modest scale. Its first year's total turnover was approximately equivalent to $40,000. As the years went by production in size and number of products and brands increased without, however, reaching a volume warranting organization into a separate division. Later, a separate sales but not manufacturing organization was set up.

From the pre-war history of Universal's household product division two facts of significance stand out. The first is that the class of trade was not particularly directed towards the higher socio-economic brackets. Yet in retrospect this is seen as an halcyon era. Among the elder members of the present-day sales force there is a persisting fantasy relating to the division's pre-war type of business. When discussing this period, phrases such as 'the best homes', 'the finest people', with obvious reference to socio-economic groups recur again and again. Clearly, this is a direct reversal of the facts, indicating at the very least that some of these men with pre-war experience in the division feel door-to-door selling to be an undignified activity.

Second, the beginning of the split between the household product and the industrial sides of this industry can be seen in the off-hand way in which the parent division treated its new subsidiary. It is clear that the production engineers of the industrial side wanted to have as little as possible to do with household products.

Immediately after the second world war a new chairman took over at Universal. During the war the capital products part of Universal had invariably suffered. It was decided to concentrate and rebuild and modernize this part of the business as a first priority. This decision, not unnatural in itself, was closely in line with national policy at the time. But shortage of key men and materials in the early post-war years delayed the completion of the task.

Several years later the chairman went to America. There he noted among other things the degree to which the household product business was advanced and on his return decided to pay greater attention to this part of the firm. The sub-division was made into a separate group with its own production facilities and its own small quantity of finance. The industrial engineers welcomed this decision. In the words of one of them it 'got household products out of our hair',

It also gave the industrial side itself a chance to obtain greater independence.

The chairman, then, looked for someone who could successfully run this newly organized division. He explained (in an interview) that:

> '[household products] are not engineering in the sense that heavy plant or [industrial] devices are, but present problems in design, styling and marketing which are peculiar to themselves . . . people who make [capital goods] are apt to carry the thinking prevailing there into other applications such as [household products]. . . . Engineers have the wrong mind for this. They look down their noses on [household products]. To them it is all bits and pieces. You can't marry this kind of thinking and engineering thinking.'

He looked for someone who could 'run the household product business, who could make a better show of it'. A short-list was arrived at. He then asked some of his closer colleagues on the Board if they knew of someone on the outside whom they could bring in for that purpose. One of the Universal's directors suggested calling in a real outsider, i.e. a non-engineering man – C. B. Alexander.

To hire him for the job represented a quite unorthodox decision. A number of people who have been all their lives in the industry cannot recall a case in the last forty-three years in which a complete outsider was entrusted with a leading managerial position in the industry. A short time later, in 1956, Mr. Alexander was appointed.

THE NEW TOP-MANAGEMENT TEAM

(a) The New Policy

Alexander took the job on condition that he was allowed to make a study of the situation for a three-to-four-month period, and then make recommendations to be accepted by Universal in principle. These would become the broad policy on which he would run the division. Among his first acts was to bring in a colleague who had worked with him for more than a decade – M. F. Joseph. This first appointment was a key one. Together they prepared the basic plan covering the division's objectives, the organization required, the resources financial and otherwise that would be needed, and the bringing in of new staff. It was specified in this plan that these new men should come from outside the industry. Essentially Alexander's survey was the application of modern methods of marketing to the specific conditions of the division.

This was an entirely new approach in this section of the industry. It is widely agreed within the company that his predecessor was a heavy-engineering man. Characteristically, he had made his headquarters at the factory in the provinces and not in the capital of the country, the place for marketing and sales. His motto is quoted as 'let them [the customers] buy and then we will make the stuff'.

Planning, at this time, appeared in some ways erratic. During a conversation with a group of his former subordinates, the following remark was made:

'Maybe he understood us better; maybe we knew him better. Maybe today things don't always go as we would like them. But we know where we are going, what we produce and in what quantities. It is so much easier by having a plan and a directive than just fretting in uncertainty.'

The factory was organized to produce small batches of a very wide range of products. The product B model (see *Table 1*) was based on a design that had not greatly changed for more than twenty years and was, in fact, American in origin. According to long-service employees the level of production was decided intuitively and the sales force was employed to sell what the factory produced.

Pre-war, the division had manufactured about 30 per cent of the product B output in the country. But in post-war years its share of the market had sadly declined. In 1948 17 per cent of all of product B found in the country's homes was of Universal make. In 1956 this figure had come down to 8 per cent, and sales for that year were expected to be no more than 5 per cent of the industry's total.

In the course of the material presented here it will become important to study the personality of Alexander. In view of this, I shall let him speak for himself at some length on the various points raised. This is to indicate not only the content but also his approach to business planning. The Alexander appraisal of the situation based itself on the premise that: 'the market is likely to continue its long-term growth . . . the general indications are that the market will grow strongly, and for some time. . . .'

The immediate objective it put forward was: 'to arrest the fall (in the division's business) and then begin building towards achieving a major and profitable share of the [household products] market for Universal.'

The means of achieving this was to be through concentration of effort. At the time, although the division made about two hundred different brands of twenty-odd different types of household product, these varied widely in marketing importance. Taking the country's total market of the twenty-odd product groups manufactured by Universal, the nine smallest represented merely 5 per cent of the total household products market. However, 70 per cent of national production in these categories was accounted for by the three largest – products B, C, and H (see *Table 1*). It was, therefore, decided to abandon minor product groups and make a maximum effort in the major product groups. The aim was:

'to achieve in certain major fields a position sufficiently dominant to give Universal a measure of control over the market. In all other fields where Universal's business seemed likely to be minor or unprofitable, the objective would be to operate only if there were strong and special advantages in doing so. . . . In the absence of special reasons Universal would forgo these in order to concentrate its resources on the more important objectives.'

Within the major product groups the decision was taken to give main priority to product B, because: 'It is the largest field; we have considerable experience in it; we probably have both trade and consumer goodwill in it; it seems likely to be profitable.'

Since the basic objective was to 'achieve a much larger share of a competitive market', this implied 'persuading a very large number of people (who then were not of this mind) that they should buy certain Universal products.' This in turn implied 'spending heavily on advertising and sales promotion directed at the consumer'. 'Such major spending could of course be undertaken on judgement alone.' But this is a hazardous and uncertain course which can lead to marketing failure and financial loss. 'The wisdom of such a decision was linked to two basic factors – quality and cost.' The questions were raised:

'(i) Is Universal's product sufficiently outstanding to deserve continuing consumer choice after the company would revert to a normal advertising expenditure?
'(ii) Is cost sufficiently low (in relation to competition and the market) to yield an adequate margin for advertising and profit, so that the company can recover the heavy investment in a reasonable time?'

As a result of the analysis of these two questions it was decided:

'not to recommend the expenditure of large sums in an early attack on the market with Universal's existing products . . . [the immediate] objective should be to consolidate [the] existing share of the market rather than attempt a hasty expansion.'

However, for future expansion a marketing policy was recommended according to which:

'(i) We must develop and improve our product until it has a clear preference over both known and predictable competition. The work of product development, and the assessment of consumer preference, must be based on reliable research as well as on our judgement.
'(ii) We must reduce both our design cost and our manufacturing cost until we are certain that we are at no cost disadvantage relative to competition. Minor cost premiums may be acceptable for major advantages in consumer appeal.'

As to investment spending it was recommended that:

'Once we have developed a product which is proved to be superior to competition, at a satisfactory low cost, then we can with confidence spend heavily on advertising, sales promotion, and selling effort, knowing that we will build and hold the business.

'The greater the amount of this investment spending, the more readily we can hope to attain a given share of a market. However, the investment must be balanced against the predictable return.'

On organization the following principles were laid down:

'All our organization thinking needs to be focused on the single aim of increasingly winning a favourable decision from the consumer. This in turn depends on two most critical factors.
(i) Product Quality, and (ii) Effective Marketing.'

A structure 'believed to be the right one for obtaining the objectives' was sketched out. This structure separated the Sales Department and the Marketing Department. The responsibility of the former was 'with their buyers – *the trade*', of the latter 'for achieving the ultimate favourable decision from *the consumer*'.

Product-planning was described in great detail as designed to create 'an outstanding product which *deserves* to be purchased', and to achieve 'an *actual* purchase by the consumer'.

As to personnel, 'have an organization of better-than-average calibre' was recommended. Conditions of employment were suggested relating to the various customary features. But this policy suggestion included 'above all, warm and enthusiastic leadership'.

The morale of the personnel at Universal had been shaken by several major reorganizations and other disturbances in the two years before Alexander came to the company. It was, therefore, decided to 'minimize further unsettling actions for the present'. This was done in the full realization that there were:

'Some positions in the organization held by people of limited ability . . . competitive success will depend on having really outstanding people in all key positions, but the necessary changes and adjustments should not be done too hastily.'

It was also recognized that: 'the cost of building a first-class organization is likely to rise faster than its fruits – so we face a period of investment-in-people.'

This plan was approved in its entirety by the Chairman and accepted by the board of Universal. Of Alexander's position henceforth, one of his colleagues has remarked:

'From that date on he had no interference from anyone as far as expenditure or employment or product development policy [were concerned]. He was *in fact* chief executive of the division, and this merely on the guarantee that he would remove a lost position and produce a healthy profit position.'

(b) The Changes Start

For the first six months very few changes were made in the actual organization of the division. The period was mainly devoted to collecting information. In Joseph's words, it appeared that 'the industry was badly off so far as statistics were concerned'. The first task, therefore, was really to find out:

'whether the recommendation was really true. We made a lot of assumptions about volume, acceptance of products and so . . . the first period of time was employed with detailed market research both statistically and in the field.'

There were, of course, also other things to do.

'For the first six months it was mainly a question of economy, because the business was badly in the red . . . of studying the market, and of trying to assess what sort of personnel were necessary in the whole field.'

Alexander's attitude towards the problem of company structure is best illustrated by the organization chart which he introduced at an early stage. Most organization charts are shaped like a family tree with the chairman and managing director at the top and the various successive levels of management and organization below them. Moreover, in the usual type of chart departments depend on other departments, so that the outer branches of the tree, as it were, are remote from each other and from the board. Alexander's chart places the managing director and his staff in the centre, with four departments – Marketing, Design, Manufacturing, and Sales – radiating out from the centre. In addition there is a symbol of how he intended to orientate the group thinking. The consumer is represented in the dominating position at the top of the chart.

The division had never had a marketing department, and during this period one was started as well as the nucleus of a market research organization.

By the end of the six-month period the new management had decided that the engineering side of the company was 'relatively strong, though not brilliant', and thus did not require immediate strengthening in the way the marketing and sales side did.

About a year later it was decided that there was a need to bring fresh blood into the designing and engineering department. By this time the division was engaged in developing new and more complicated products, and, therefore, started a vigorous recruiting campaign for designers and engineers, although the actual number involved was not large.

A beginning was also made in engaging new staff both for marketing and sales. Many of the new men, particularly in marketing, came from one or other of the companies with which the new management has been associated. This happened for two reasons. The men knew Alexander and his method of work, and they came from companies which had been operating in highly competitive markets and whose marketing techniques had proved to be very efficient. Moreover, by agreeing to move with Alexander to Universal, these men were demonstrating in the most practical manner a high degree of loyalty and confidence in his leadership.

At the same time a conscious attempt was made to gain

the confidence and good will of older members of the staff – especially in the sales force – some of whom had been with the company for twenty years and more. Not unnaturally, the upheaval had caused a great deal of anxiety among them. Even three years after this period, when the author discussed with some of these men their feelings at the time, they reproduced vividly their anxieties of that time. As the new team gathered around Alexander, the older members of the staff felt increasingly outsiders. They found it difficult to believe that a man who was new to the job and the industry and whose methods appeared alien to tradition would be a success. To some extent, it appears, they even held back technical knowledge they possessed, ostensibly in order not to offend. As one long-standing staff member said: 'To contradict the managing director was to commit *lèse-majesté*. So it was best to leave him be.'

The management attempted to overcome this apparent resistance by showing the staff results that the market research department was producing. The purpose of this was to convince them that the new models being developed would be acceptable to the public and that, therefore, sales targets could be introduced successfully. These efforts, however, met with great scepticism. As one of these men put it to the author: 'We hoped that the new management would go away like a bad dream.'

For the first time in their experience systematic training of the sales force was introduced. There was follow-up training and each salesman was given a target to attain. The aim was to make the sales force regard itself as salesmen, not travellers, since in the words of an executive 'their function was to sell and not to travel around making a series of social calls'. The change in approach was from 'making a call to ask: "Do you want anything today?" to putting forward reasons why the buyer should obtain the products'. As the company expanded its business, scepticism turned to unwilling recognition of success. One old-timer said:

'Damned if I know why we are so successful. [These] products have a snob value, they are not a necessity. My mother never had [these new-fangled things], but maybe she is old-fashioned like me. She wouldn't have it as a present. The reason for the success escapes me. Frankly, it often shakes me. There are so many changes in this company, I would not know where to begin.'

A system of small premium prizes was introduced. League tables were drawn up and individual and collective prizes awarded. A salesman would be called in and politely asked the reason why an account had not bought any of the products in question. The man might reply that the dealer was overstocked. But after twenty-five or more similar replies, this answer, as a sales executive expressed it, 'wears thin'. By the end of this relentless inquisition the point had been made clear to the salesman. This method, it is said, effected an amazing improvement in results. There can be no doubt that some of this improvement must be attributed to the anxiety it induced in the salesman.

The increased efficiency of the sales force is shown by the following statistics. In August 1956 the total sales force consisted of fifty men. On 1 January 1960, by which time sales of the company had been multiplied several times over, there were still only sixty-seven salesmen, thirty-eight of whom were members of the old sales force. Only two of the original team lost their jobs; the other ten were accounted for by transfers or natural wastage.

Meanwhile an important step had been taken by introducing what were known as 'procedure books'. The purpose was to plot in the utmost detail what each department and each person had to do at any stage. They included a check-

83

back form to make sure the procedure was being complied with. Thus the procedure had two purposes. One was to provide a detailed job specification, which not merely let each person know exactly what he was doing but also compelled the managers to work out whether each particular person or operation was really needed. Second, the checkback form could be used in the next promotion or trade campaign in order to make sure that the lesson of experience was learned. As Joseph put it:

'Put on top of the list [of changes] having detailed plans and procedures of exactly how we should operate, instead of people operating by rule of thumb. I don't mean by that that we had procedure books that you must arrive by 9 o'clock in the morning. But we had procedure books for launching a new product. These are the 52 steps the company will take which are divided between all the departments of the company and they'll be cleared and checked in every instance, so that care was taken to avoid making mistakes and to launch programmes according to date schedules.'

The next stage was to carry out the decision to limit the company's range of products. One executive stated: 'Universal had the widest range of household products, more than any other competitor. Then started concentration on more important product groups.'

It was decided in particular to abandon a great deal of commercial and industrial business. Besides concentrating resources and manpower, this enabled the new team to exploit what they regarded as their particular skill – selling to the consumer.

As far as selling policy was concerned, the major change was a decision to concentrate as far as possible on dealing directly with the retailer. Before 1956, Universal operated largely through wholesalers at the ratio of 70 per cent wholesaler sales to 30 per cent direct retailer sales. Apart from the question of the wholesale margin it was felt that direct retail business offered two advantages. There was more chance of directing the selling operation, since the company would be dealing directly with the shopkeeper who had to do the selling, and Universal's own sales force would have the opportunity to stand on the shop floor and demonstrate. As part of this policy, retailers were given a degree of preference in deliveries. The company insisted that to enjoy wholesale discounts wholesalers would have to perform a full wholesaling function by actually carrying stock and ordering in quantities. If they attempted only to order what they sold, they were treated as retailers and charged retail prices.

This policy, not unexpectedly, caused antagonism on the part of the wholesale distributors. There was an attempted boycott which, however, lasted only three months and then broke down. A more serious difficulty was that the same wholesaler bought other products of other divisions of Universal and thus for a time there was some internal upset. However, these difficulties were smoothed out. Within three years three-quarters of the division's business was conducted directly through retailers, and it is worth noting that many of its competitors who had not already 'gone retail' had decided to follow suit.

Finally, there remains the change made in the advertising approach. In view of the difference between the product C and product B markets, it is important to make separate analyses of Universal's advertising campaigns for these two product groups. The most important fact about the product C market during the years 1958 and 1959 was that for the industry as a whole demand was considerably in excess of supply. Thus, very largely, manufacturers' market shares

FIGURE 1 — HOUSEHOLD PRODUCT B

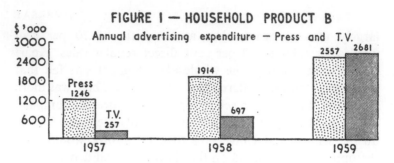

Annual advertising expenditure — Press and T.V.

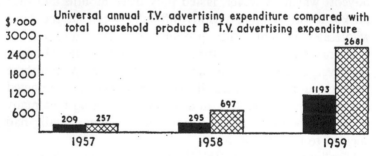

Universal annual T.V. advertising expenditure as percentage of total household product B T.V. advertising expenditure

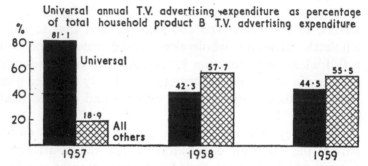

Universal annual T.V. advertising expenditure compared with total household product B T.V. advertising expenditure

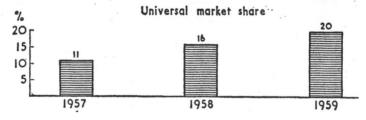

Universal market share

FIGURE 2 — HOUSEHOLD PRODUCT C

Annual advertising expenditure — Press and T.V.

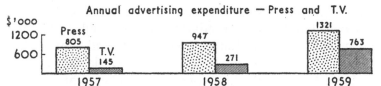

Universal annual T.V. advertising expenditure as percentage of total household product C T.V. advertising expenditure

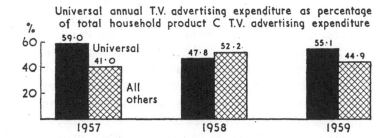

Universal annual T.V. advertising expenditure compared with total household product C T.V. advertising expenditure

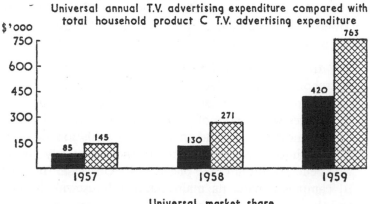

Universal market share

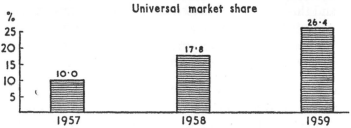

were determined by the rate at which they produced and by the availability of their products. *Figures 1* and *2* show the manufacturers' expenditure on advertising and their market shares in these two years. However, since availability was the main problem during this period, it would be unsafe to draw any firm conclusions about the effectiveness of Universal's advertising either by itself or compared to that of its competitors. It does seem, however, that there is no obvious direct connection between the volume of advertising and the market shares of the various companies in this field.

During this period Universal combined heavy advertising with the launching of new products. Its advertising campaign was inaugurated in three different ways. First, in sheer volume of expenditure, as can be seen from an inspection of *Figures 1* and *2*. Much of the rest of the industry followed suit. Secondly, in the content of the advertising, which a director of its agency has described in this way:

'Up to the time of Universal's new management, all household product advertising was very much manufacture orientated. Advertisements promoted the product and its features with a note of pride in the manufacturing and design know-how behind them. The translation of these features into consumer benefit – or more precisely housewife benefit – did not take place ... the Universal [product B] campaign made its main claim a housewife benefit, and this benefit was presented in a very concentrated and, we believe, effective manner. The temptation to try and tell the housewife everything about the product with the inevitable result of registering nothing, was firmly resisted.'

Basically, the strategy was to use one particular 'housewife benefit' as the main point of advertisement. No other manufacturer had made use of a single product difference in this way up till then. Increasingly, from 1958 onwards, the copy of other product B manufacturers appeared influenced by this approach. Some of Universal's competitors went so far as to specifically adopt the particular 'housewife benefit' mentioned above.

Third, there was a very marked departure in the use of advertising media. Previously expenditure had been spread fairly evenly over a variety of media. Universal's new management and its agency decided that since the ideal way to sell a product B would be actually to present it in the home, the nearest approach to this in advertising could be provided by television. Consequently, from the very beginning there was an increasing concentration on television advertising. In 1959 Universal spent nearly three times as much on television as on press advertising.

(c) The Results begin to Show

The results of the new policy can be seen most clearly in *Table 2* below.

TABLE 2. PRODUCT B – UNIVERSAL FORECAST IN 1956 AND ACTUAL SALES (The figures represent percentages)*

	Total market		Universal market share	
Year	Forecast	Actual	Forecast	Actual
1957	100	120·5	12	11
1958	125	173·75	16	18
1959	150	270·0	20	20

*The figures are expressed in percentages and not in actual numbers at the request of Universal.

A number of points emerge from the study of *Table 2*:

1. It will be seen that over the period of three years Universal's share of the product B market rose from

89

11 per cent to 18 per cent to 20 per cent. Comparing this with the forecast made in 1956, there is an amazingly close correspondence.

2. The 1956 forecast of how the total market would grow is shown to be a very serious underestimate. This is presumably because in 1956 it was impossible to foresee that all instalment-purchase controls would be removed two years later.

3. Although the total market grew much faster than had been anticipated, Universal was able to expand its own production to keep pace with it. This is a considerable achievement and casts a favourable light not only on the company's flexibility but also on the quality of its organization.

It would be wrong to attribute this success merely to the introduction of new products. There was an equally striking success in increasing the sales of an old model that had been in production since the early 1930's and the design of which had not been changed by the new team. Extensive use was made of market research in designing another model. In 1958, the first year of its production, it took nearly 20 per cent of its total product group market; in 1959 nearly one third. As Alexander said:

'Universal, prior to this management, was not exploiting their share of the market, which it should have done. To that extent we had a couple of rosy apples dropped in our hands. The public acceptance of the product was there, but the old management was not using it.'

Although, as has been indicated, the main effort was concentrated on product B, other Universal products shared to some extent in the improvement. Taking the country as a whole, there was in 1959 an increase of 35 per cent over the previous year on the amount spent by the public on household products. Universal's sales were 55 per cent higher. Its output of product B was doubled in 1958 and again in 1959, product B sales were 65 per cent higher in 1959, while among other products the introduction of a product G proved a considerable success.

As a result, the level of net profit which the original plan had foreseen would be reached towards the end of the 1960s was in fact achieved in 1959. Admittedly, the complete abandonment of instalment-purchase restrictions made 1959 a uniquely favourable year. But the company went steadily ahead in the widely varying conditions of the previous two years. It appears to be dealing far more realistically than most of its competitors with the difficulties created by the subsequent reimposition of instalment-purchase restrictions. Moreover, 1959 showed for Universal an increased share of a highly competitive market.

(d) Attitudes of the Division's Management

Since the shape of the new Universal policy was determined essentially by its managing director, C. B. Alexander, and his aide Joseph, it is the attitudes of these two men which are described and discussed in the following section.

(i) *Forward planning.* In discussing the non-leader companies it was possible to make a sharp distinction between their executives' attitudes to the consumer, to the market, and to the distributor. This was feasible because of the incisive and almost total separation of these subjects in the interviewees' minds. When discussing the attitudes of the Universal management to the same subjects, no such division proved possible, since, for reasons which will appear later, the three topics proved to be fused in the minds of those concerned.

Basically the trade, wholesalers and dealers, are regarded as 'channels of distribution' through which Universal aims

91

to reach through to the consumer. Alexander defined the task as:

> '. . . strong advertisement and considerable improvement in our standard of salesmanship into the trade and of our sales demonstrators, helping the trade selling to the public, coupled in the usual way with merchandizing and promotion.'

So far, therefore, from being the 'be all and end all' of business to be approached with respect by the sales force, dealers are regarded as frankly needing help. They are useful, they help to reach the public, they deserve support in that respect. One gets the impression that at least some of the dealers are not considered quite grown up in the circumstances of today, i.e. 'they have not yet understood nor accepted the modern marketing principle'.

On forward planning, Alexander regards marketing as a key to the whole situation. He said:

> '. . . the marketing department . . . was not alone and primarily the reason for our share of the market. But in the steering and directing of our organizational activities, I would give it a very high place in a causative way . . . the Marketing Department is the source of dynamic co-ordination to the whole of our business.'

Alexander believes in marketing with a quasi-religious fervour that finds its expression in repeated use of the phrase 'dynamic co-ordination'. It appears sometimes as 'consumer-orientated dynamic co-ordination'.

Also, and in contrast to the non-leader executives, he evinces confidence in and readiness to make use of the full apparatus of market research. In particular he pins his faith on the rational use of sales forecasting. Joseph describes this by saying:

'Alexander worked for a [foreign] company for twenty-two years and I was with them only for eight years. They were particularly hot on forecasting. . . . It is the management's willingness to accept forecasting. It is reasonably easy when it is good. But when it differs in personal judgement that's where I think the strength of management comes in. I know of several instances when managements say we must have market research. But, then, when it is good they buy it and when it is bad they tend to ignore it.'

It is worth noting at this point that the head of marketing at Universal sits on the board of the company, is in continuous contact with the managing director, and had helped to write the original policy brief. Thus, he does not merely see to the analysis and evaluation of marketing data but is also in a state of continuous alertness to the opportunities suggested by the data. His is essentially a policy-shaping role, as Alexander recognizes when he says: 'He helps me to think.' This is in marked difference to the non-leader companies, where those which have market research departments, which are by no means all, accord them only a junior status. Their heads have no part in policy and are often unaware of what the policy is. They merely collect data and pass them on. Most of the non-leader companies have no marketing department at all.

In further contrast to the non-leaders' attitudes of resignation, almost fatalism, Alexander and Joseph display a high degree of ambition. In reply to the question: 'What does the term *the market* really mean?', Joseph replied seriously:

'The only thing that we exclude from the market is the moon and Mars, which, I believe, are the only two likely places that people will go to in this century, if the Russian kind of forecasting is right. I wasn't trying to be facetious.

I mean this seriously. We regard the whole world as our market.'

More concretely, they are determined, till such time as rockets are perfected, to make an attack on markets overseas. In Alexander's words:

'I have a very strong view on this. It has been a painful view to persist in the easy markets in [this country], but I am quite certain that we must be out there building a large business in the overseas market. Not only in export but, in due course, in overseas assembly and, in the long run, in overseas manufacture. I see a trend towards greater flow, greater trade between countries, tariff barriers coming down, easier travel, better transport, and all the rest of it. I don't think that one can say that while we have our share of the home market, we don't have to worry about all these things; they don't speak our language and we've got to get salesmen who speak [other language], so we just get on in our own market. You may do so for five, ten, or fifteen years, but in the long run someone is going to be much bigger than you in the international market wherever they are, that his costs are going to be substantially lower. I think the climate of the world opinion is going to be against the enormous tariff barriers and so, I believe, in the long run, if you are going to compete in the home market or anywhere else, you must be prepared to compete in the world. For that reason we have . . . put a lot of effort into building up from almost scratch in the beginning, and it is no more than the most elementary beginning yet. It is an attack on the major markets of the world.'

(ii) *Product planning*. Alexander's emphasis on marketing shows perhaps at its clearest in his attitude to product planning. On this subject he says:

'. . . you command success only if you are offering to the

94

customer something which is better than she has been able to buy up to then. This primarily comes back to product. But the finest product in the world won't get bought unless the customer knows about it and knows why it is a fine product. An outstanding product coupled with strong advertising, strong merchandizing, strong display and strong selling in any field in the retail outlet; these are the basic things. I would not begin to spend money against advertising and sales effort and anything else until we have the right product. I think if there is one thing that perhaps we have been uniquely insistent on is that we will not go to the market until we are absolutely certain about a product. Now this makes it late for the market. We could have gone to the market much earlier with something hastily designed, hastily produced and we could have had a lot of trouble with it. On balance, this is something that I am not willing to risk. So we have a little saying: "We don't want to be first in the market, we just want to be best." This is something which we feel very deeply.'

The key to this passage is not the insistence on a perfect product, but the definition of perfection in terms of being right for the market. He goes on:

'. . . the product superiority is achieved largely by a marketing approach. And to that extent marketing is critical in achieving the product. But there are a lot of people with quite good marketing and marketing team in their companies who don't have this emphasis on product. This is one of the very few things which I do not delegate . . . the final yea or nay on product characteristics . . . product is so critical in my judgement . . . I want to play awfully personally and awfully closely. Because, unless you have the right product, all this investment and all the marketing thinking will lead you nowhere.'

95

Clearly the production engineer is no longer king. He is being used, guided, and directed in an effort to get to the consumer. The remark of the non-leader executive who said:

'You see how many advantages this model [product F] has? From an engineer's point of view it is as good as can be manufactured for the market. But do housewives buy it as they should?'

can be contrasted with Alexander's reply to the researcher stating: 'your technical people are not that much better than other technical men in this country'. He answered:

'Probably not. In some areas we would like to think that we are a little better. But by and large we have no great overall superiority. But what is important is to guide that technical work into the correct channel productwise.'

There is no doubt in Alexander's mind that the needs of the market are the guide for the purpose.

(iii) *Advertising*. The management's attitude to advertising appears to be as straightforward as are its attitudes to the trade and the engineering side of the business. It is neither a fetish nor a whipping boy but something to be used as a means of getting to the public. Alexander said:

'I don't think advertising without real product differences will help you very much, if you haven't got a real product advantage which you are talking about in your advertising and which you are talking about in a *believable* way, which is also important.'

In accordance with the primacy that he gives to marketing, as opposed to production or selling, he defines the necessary order of action as first developing and exploiting product advantages, as defined above, and then proceeding to advertise heavily. Joseph stated:

'. . . up to 1956, the average level of expenditure on advertising was 1½ per cent of net sales of all [household products]. We had been launching products, starting off with 10 per cent of sales figures and coming down on a going basis to something like 5 per cent. Some of the major people left us alone to do that for six months or nine months; as soon as they found that the boot pinched, they rapidly started to boost their own advertising. There are a number of people in the business who spend three and four times the level they used to two and three years back, and this must increase and widen the market considerably.'

(iv) *Selling*. Selling, to Alexander and Joseph, means largely pre-selling through getting the right product, marketing, and advertising. Thus the sales force itself, though regarded as important, was not accorded for a long time particularly senior status. One of the sales executives stated: 'To pay salesmen more [than the equivalent of $3,000 per annum] is morally wrong.'

Other signs of the comparatively lower status have been a certain chopping and changing in the management of the selling side, with three different sales directors in three years. This indicates that, as far as the sales force was concerned, the new management perpetuated to some extent attitudes that are common throughout the rest of the industry. It seems that the new team achieved its success in spite of the lower status its sales force had. It would be legitimate to conjecture that a more positive attitude to the sales force might have made the success of the company still greater.

In fairness it must be said that there were signs of a change of attitude on this issue towards the end of the period

97

covered by this study. A start was made on strengthening the sales organization. In part, however, this comes from a recognition on the top management's part that the sales force, as one of its needs, has been seeking status. The change takes the form of greater willingness to grant this than hitherto.

(v) *Household Products.* In describing the attitudes of Universal's top-level management to household products, the following dialogue is worth quoting in full:

AUTHOR: What I particularly would like to ask you: what, in your opinion, does a [household product] stand for in [this country]?

ALEXANDER: What does it stand for? I do not know exactly what it stands for. You mean why do they buy them?

AUTHOR: Well, in addition to utilitarian purposes, what else does a [household product] fulfil?

ALEXANDER: Of course, obviously, it has a considerable prestige value. It stands for having something worth while, satisfaction. For instance, the first time a husband can afford to buy his wife a [product B]. In the [national] market, of course, we are at the stage where the majority of homes still don't have these things. I am sure that in addition to the sheer logical and practical usefulness of the thing there is a much bigger sense of achievement and satisfaction. The right of possession in the minds of the buyer. I think this a very right and proper feeling in a man's mind or in a housewife's mind, that she wants or that he wants his wife and family to have – a useful and helpful [product C].

The first point to note about this interchange is that in contrast to the non-leader executives' nearly unanimous discussion of household products in terms of lightening the housewife's burden, Alexander sees them in largely emotional terms – satisfaction and something worth while. Note too, that the example he gives of satisfaction is 'the first time a husband can afford to buy his wife a [product B]'. This example might not seem significant, if it were not that the non-leader executives at no time mentioned the family situation or the role of the husband. Secondly, it is worth noting from the point of view of the company management team that there is a contrast between Alexander's warm emotionalism and Joseph's reserve, almost complete absence of emotional overtones bordering on embarrassment. When asked: 'What do household products really mean, what do they stand for?', Joseph replied:

'We understand by a [household product] any product which might be used in the home. We deliberately turned our back on a lot of industrial business for shops or for hotels, stuff of that sort, to concentrate on the consumer market.'

This expresses a rapid switch from the area of emotion, i.e. potential embarrassment, to an objective discussion on a business technique.

(vi) *Government policies and regulations.* The Universal management appears to be unique among the major household product firms in that it has little or no commitment to the defence of resale price maintenance. It was the author's impression that Alexander was out of sympathy with the line of argument put forward by certain bodies in favour of resale price maintenance. Whatever the merits of their case as applied to their own field, he felt that the interests of the public at large, as opposed to those of a particular group of manufacturers, were of overriding importance, and that government policy should, and no doubt would, be guided by the wider considerations.

His general attitude in short, again in contrast to the non-leaders, is a recognition that on this issue he is not a technical expert and that other interests may well have priority over the particular interest in his firm. It appeared to be his view that it was wrong for the big buyer to be free to use his power to secure particularly favourable trading terms, which, in turn, enable him to become bigger and more monopolistic. Although he felt he was not an expert on the technical issues involved, he was inclined to support legislation such as the Robinson-Patman Act in the U.S.A., whose object was to make such activities illegal.

More generally, on the question of the various government regulations such as instalment-purchase control, sales taxes, credit restrictions, etc. Alexander took the attitude that it is not fair on the part of the government to use the household products industry as the residuary legatee of national prosperity, i.e. the last to be de-restricted and the first to be controlled. On the other hand, in sharp contrast to the general attitude in the industry, he does not regard government control as a reason or excuse for fatalism or bad performance.

(vii) *Competitors.* As far as competitors are concerned there is a feeling, frankly, of considerable superiority towards them. In reply to the question: 'How do your competitors look by comparison?', Joseph said: 'There are one or two who are very efficient, there are one or two who are medium, and there are quite a lot who, in our view, are very inefficient indeed.'

Over the past two years some types of household products have been in inadequate supply relative to the demand. Alexander makes it clear that he considered the market share of his company to have been limited by production, whereas in the case of his competitors only the general shortage enabled them to sell all they made. He says:

'Whereas other manufacturers have had a sharp increase in their stock in the trade, in our case, we have almost not got any, and other cases diminished our stock in the trade. In other words everything we make is still going out by and large to the customers. The other chaps are not doing this to quite the same extent. There is some evidence, particularly on [product C] in the last year, that in the brief period in which we were in free supply, we were enjoying a market share about three times what we were able to command in the rest of the year. So that our share of market is not necessarily a true indication of the business we have built and could capture if we had the product.'

This is confirmed by Joseph who states that:

'If we had twice the capacity of all other people, I think X [competitor] would have lost a share. Assuming that we had additional capacity over and beyond the consumer demand in the last three years, Y [competitor] and Z [competitor] would have been the people who would have lost shares. Now this industry had definitely underproduced for the last three years. We were quite sure whoever had, could sell all they could make.'

The suggestion underneath this – justified or not – is that Universal, through its reliance on the religion of marketing, is able to take cognizance of and can master the external set of circumstances, while the other companies, lacking this, find their performances determined by factors outside their control.

(viii) *General attitudes*. Both Alexander and Joseph share a common basic attitude to their purpose in life. In Joseph's words:

'To me the most exciting thing in life is my work. To my boss it is the most important thing in his life. I think this is not due to a consideration to acquire money or due to a consideration to acquire position. But we both happen to enjoy working and working together, too. We have tried to choose senior people who have got the same feeling that their work is important to them, not to the extent that they become bores and have no outside interests, but the work is number one, but if there is a decision between home and work then the home always wins. There are not a lot of people who are like that. There are one or two here, at all levels; this makes an enormous difference to the amount of work done. If people are intelligent enough and work, you just get physically through a lot of work. It is almost mathematically as long as you keep the pressure up you can never be passed, like the Russian rocket, except for a mistake that no one can foresee.'

It is relevant at this point to note that Alexander, like his father, is an elder of his church. This fact determines many of his basic business activities. Success comes only to those who deserve it; there must be no short cuts, and one deserves success by hard work, diligence, acceptance of responsibility towards oneself and others, particularly those in the immediate environment. Alexander refers to 'a happy sense of where we are going and being worthy in what we are doing. A sense of being useful and productive and helpful members of the community'. A little later he remarked:

'I have a fundamental belief that anyone who undertakes the responsibility of managing other people, undertakes, whether he likes it or not, an almost sacred responsibility to do his best with their personal development. Now when we take in a young man from the university or the shop floor or wherever you like, his immediate manager and those above have a very strong and almost

102

religious responsibility to help that young man to develop and to become the best kind of person that he can. Next to that young man's wife, shall we say, we are almost the most important influence in his life, as he spends eight hours a day, or whatever it is, working. If his boss encourages him to cheat, or take short cuts, or if his boss encourages him to be slothful or any other unworthy thing, he is failing to help that chap to develop the way he should and to become a bigger, finer, more competent, and more worthy person. Now I have quite a deep feeling about this.'

It is fair to say that the phrases 'fundamental belief' and 'deep feeling' point to Alexander's *daimon*. At whatever remove, this is an expression of an essentially religious view of life. At another stage, Alexander remarked:

'. . . One of the things which above all would keep me sitting here . . . is the team that I am working with, the organization. As long as chaps like [Joseph] and [others] . . . [are] going on with it and look towards me to go on with it, I would think awfully hard about pulling out . . . there is no money that would make me pull out.'

Describing how he selects his staff, Alexander cites four basic qualities he looks for: character, personality, energy, and brains. Character he defines significantly as 'the moral qualities', because 'it is basic that you've got to be able to trust a fellow'. Personality he defined as the social qualities, warmth, friendliness, and in particular, liking of people. On energy he says:

'Now of course, you like him to be a powerhouse of energy, at least of a pretty high level of energy. He mustn't be slothful and lazy and he must show all the related qualities of rather enjoying a struggle, a battle and all the rest of it.'

It is worth noting the biblical or religious implication of his choice of the word 'slothful'. Brain he puts last. He says: 'I would never recruit a man [only] because he had an outstanding brain.'

He goes on:

'I have a very strong view on this and that is that people should be happy in their work. If they are not happy in their work, then there is something directly wrong either with the person in the job or that he is in the wrong job, or with his management. And one of the things that I like to look at very closely, when I go around the organization, the factory, the offices, the departments here and everywhere is, are people happy in their work? You get the feeling that they are enjoying the achievement and accomplishment. They can go home on Friday night tired by all means, but at least feeling we have made some progress this week, I have had some fun and we have solved a couple of problems. So, I have a nice rest and I start on Monday morning ready for the fray again.'

Finally, the stress on non-economic motives is shown very clearly in Alexander's discussion of the method for dealing with inadequate or unsatisfactory long-service staff. In reply to a question on this point he said:

'I believe that management has a very deep human responsibility for people whom the business has accepted and has had around for some years and who may have been adequate ten years ago, or even five years ago when the business was small and not particularly efficient but who are no longer adequate today. Now that does not mean that you turn around and push them out or even that you demote them ruthlessly and without thought and care. But it does mean that you recognize that old Joe is not the fellow for the next promotion and is not even good to

104

hold down his present job. Then you start worrying about how you get him out of there without killing your responsibility to him as a responsible employer. This takes time. It may take a year, or two years. We have right now several of the types of managers of whom we just know we will have to make a change and we are very worried about it. We don't see today the openings. But any time that the opportunity for change in the organization occurs, we say: "Now can we fit him into there?" We tried this one last week, but then no, this wasn't it. So we had to go along with it for a bit longer. Because you have a conflict there of setting these very high standards, at the same time you need not throw out or be ruthless with your people. In some of the places where we appear to have accepted second grade or even third grade management, it isn't because we are not planning a change, it is because we have not yet found the graceful way to make the change, the responsible way to make the change.'

Once again, one can notice that Alexander's quest for business efficiency is influenced and modified by his personal attitude.

(e) The Role of the Chief Executive

Alexander considers that the role of the chief executive has four fundamental aspects. First, deciding the structure of the organization; second, getting the right people into the right jobs; third, having given a broad outline, delegating as thoroughly as possible; and fourth, giving himself time to think. In his own words:

'And this, I am sure, is critical. And it is my aim to have something of the order of 50 per cent of my time free of all routine and day to day business so that I can think. I don't mean I sit in an ivory tower and think. I think with

105

Joseph about our future. I think about markets. I usually think with people, but this is forward-looking thinking.'

One of the most important functions of the chief executive, Alexander considers, is to

'. . . accept the fundamental responsibility, in there, pitching for profits for his shareholders. Now, if he doesn't want to do that, he must get out. If he does not want to do that, he stays under false pretences and he is cheating the shareholders. Now, I have a very strong view on that. We have a responsibility, if you like a moral responsibility, not to cheat these people who have invested their money, and they trust us to do the best with it . . . because some people have asked us if we will undertake the responsibility of trying to make profits for them, and we managers have said yes, we are going to keep our words, naturally.'

Again, there is the interplay of personal moral motives with the more objective business drive. This comes out still more strongly when he goes on to say:

'In addition to that, I hope we can do a lot more things. I hope we can personally, and that means me, and the team, have the satisfaction of accomplishment and achievement of a job well done. Of having something worthwhile, and having made a contribution to the progress of the economy. Of having, I hope, a large and growing body of satisfied customers who feel good about us because we made them fine products and gave them good value. A happy sense, if you like, of where we are going and being worthy and productive and helpful members of the community.'

At this stage two comments only need to be made on this

106

passage. First, the sense of identification between the firm and the individual. 'I hope we can personally, and that means me . . .' is a vividly revealing, although unconscious expression. Second, the sense of identification on a larger scale with the customers, so that he, his team, the company and its customers all merge into one 'worthy, useful, productive, and helpful' union. This suggests – to put it no more strongly at this point – a deep felt need to be accepted and to be respected by himself and by the community by proving that he is useful in a worthy way. It is interesting to note that the form of 'service' he has chosen throughout his business career has been to the consumer in general and to the housewife in particular, i.e. to make life easier for her with better household products. The psychological significance of this attitude will be discussed later in this study.

THE MIDDLE AND LOWER LEVELS OF THE UNIVERSAL ORGANIZATION

In studying the non-leader companies, one of their main features was shown to be the degree to which attitudes held by the top management were shared all the way down throughout the hierarchy of the company. Thus, it was possible to use the attitudes as the means of classifying the material. The situation in Universal proved to be very different. There was much less homogeneity, particularly in the marketing and sales departments of the company. Moreover, the key factor proved to be not the attitudes held by personnel to, for example, the consumer or the system of distribution, but the groups into which the staff naturally formed itself and the degree of identification between these groups and the top management. Thus, any discussion of Universal must necessarily be in terms of these groups. The sales and marketing personnel at Universal were found to be divided each into three fairly sharply defined and fairly sharply competitive groups.

(a) The Marketing Department

The marketing department, at the time of this study directly led by Joseph, was in a sense the new management's chosen instrument. This is not unnatural, since Alexander's personal experience and apparent predilection favour this approach. Attention was concentrated on marketing, and to some extent the selling side was regarded as of secondary importance when compared to marketing. This has found its symptomatic expression in repeated changes of management in the sales department, while marketing has remained continuously under its original head. One result of this can be seen in the rivalry prevailing between the two sections in the jockeying for status in the company.

All the personnel in the marketing department came to the company in 1956 or later. Thus, none has been in its employ for more than four years. Among them, however, the following clearly defined groups are to be found. The first is the original nucleus, which was engaged in the early stages. The great majority of these had worked with Alexander at one time or another in the past. These men are often wryly referred to by their colleagues as 'the apostles'. It should be noted here that the Chairman of the company is frequently called 'the father', and this widely throughout the various Universal divisions.

There are signs of the beginnings of a 'private and symbolic language' among this group of men, used among themselves and in contact with Alexander, the terms of which are drawn from the language of sailing. Phrases such as 'it's in the boat', 'getting its sea legs', 'sit at the helm', 'ballast', abound. This is an obvious emulation of the chief executive, whose personal hobby is yachting. When discussing a new sales campaign, the meeting was opened with a quote from Alexander which he had made at another meeting.

'The weather has been fair as far as the industry as a whole was concerned. We, therefore, made good progress. But it is not in fact until we run into heavy weather, that the crew is really tested, and it is possible then to check whether they've been properly trained and whether their outlook is right.'

Significantly, members of the newer group at this meeting expressed their optimism by remarks such as – 'it's in the boat' and 'full speed ahead', while some of the men who had been with the company before the advent of the new management spoke of 'walking the plank'.

There are even indications of an earlier 'private language' based on the terms of the art of advertising. This has been noticed on the highest level; the chairman remarked: 'Alexander and his boys have always dealt with consumers. They even have a language of their own.'

Among the main features of this group are their deeply felt loyalty, amounting almost to hero-worship, to the chief executive, apparent freedom of access to him whenever it is desired and – perhaps enhanced by the process of identi-fication – a close identity of thought with him and each other. Most of these men are university graduates like Alexander himself.

Another group in the marketing department came to the company about eighteen months later, that is, sometime in 1958. There are fewer college graduates among them, and they were in general from a lower echelon of management. Owing to this second group's less senior position, they naturally find it less easy to gain access to the chief executive and have to use their superiors as channels. One finds among them hero-worship but also frustration, together with a degree of envy of their superiors, i.e. the original nucleus. They seem to feel that their progress depends on direct contact with the top management and without it they are deprived of effectiveness. This frustration, leading to ambivalence, finds its expression in the form of a sometimes personal resentment towards Alexander shown fairly clearly in the following three statements:

'I love my boss. I love what he is doing. I believe in it. This is no build-up. But when he is not in, the shop is freer and easier. . . . But I stay here because I believe in what he is doing. There are enough jobs around, so that I do not have to be here.'

'Alexander and Joseph are the finest men I ever worked for. At times they make mistakes, sometimes real blunders. But they always admit them. Where else do you find this?'

'We are all new to [this business]. By comparison I am only five minutes in this business. At times, I wonder whether we know what we are doing. But there is always enthusiasm, team work, a fine spirit, and we are getting places. You can ascribe it all to Alexander and of course to Joseph.'

Admiration, partly grudging and partly unfeigned, is shown particularly in the following remark: 'Alexander has the attitude of the Pilgrim Fathers, live frugally and work hard. But he is dynamic. He creates and helps us to create opportunities for ourselves.'

One reason why anxiety in this group is intensified is the fact that Alexander himself achieved success early in life, becoming a director of another company at the age of twenty-eight. Among the respondents in this group there were five men, all of whom expressed fears that age might rob them of their ambition of becoming chief executive of the division themselves. They were all in their early thirties.

The third group which can be distinguished in the marketing department consists of more recent arrivals, both recruits and trainees, but particularly the latter, all of whom have come from universities, with an emphasis on this country's equivalent of the Ivy League in America. A higher proportion of this group and indeed all the trainees have university degrees. In this respect they resemble the first group described here but are unlike the middle group, which was recruited much more on the basis of varied practical experience. Among the new arrivals and, most particularly, among the trainees a dominant attitude is one of resentment expressed in distaste for the company. They carefully cultivate an attitude of superiority to the non-college men who train them, to the job itself, and to the atmosphere of the company. One of them remarked to the author:

'You should have seen our last sales conference. It was loud, vulgar, even distasteful. But I suppose this is how you sell effectively. Well, I can learn it, but I do not have to let it corrupt me personally.'

In part this is no more than an expression of insecurity in the form of insistence on inflated self-importance. One trainee said:

'The best brains in the country are to be found at the universities. We are the elite of the country. We carefully selected our job after interviewing various companies. Today we can afford to do this.'

Behind this naïve conceit, however, there is another and more fundamental attitude. It would be a mistake to think that this group is immune from hero-worship of the chief executive. In fact, they were attracted to Universal because

111

of its reputation. As one said: 'We took Universal not because we liked it but because we thought we could learn the new technique [marketing] here best. We will give the company two years of ourselves.'

Another one said: 'It is really a perfect jumping-board to be able to say: I have been with Alexander. This is a passport.' In other words, they see themselves in a couple of years going out as the new Alexanders to meet a greatly increased demand for trained marketing experts.

In reality, however, they have no access to their 'idol'. They are trained by people who are themselves frustrated by the difficulty of access and they feel that they are not given responsible jobs. The chief executive himself appears quite unaware of these attitudes. When given evidence of these attitudes, although in a carefully formulated, non-identifiable way, his response was: 'Really? An almost distaste? . . . Well, I am very interested and a little surprised and a little taken aback.'

Then 'thinking aloud' as he put it, he went on:

'. . . I think, inevitably that these young men from universities, from seats of higher learning, are a little sceptical, a little critical of the practical. This is not necessarily a condemnation of these young men. Because you see it in every generation of them, every year, of them having a little difficulty in making the adjustment towards this 'sordid' business of earning a living, as distinct from the elegant business of getting an education.'

While there may be some support for this view, nevertheless it does suggest a reluctance to seriously consider the possibility of the existence of a disaffected group. When the author suggested that there was deep affection towards the chief executive in the first and second groups, he replied: 'I don't know, I think you over-emphasize the part that I

112

play in this thing. Because there are the same people down the line. I know for instance that Joseph, his people have a tremendous . . .'

This statement sounds ambiguous, even contradictory. While consciously Alexander refused to accept the hypothesis of his importance to his staff, he implies the acceptance of this by suggesting that the same thing applies to Joseph. He then goes on to say:

'. . . there is wonderful personal support. This is the most priceless thing in the world to me and I think to anybody. But if we do a good job in selecting the chaps at the intermediate level, then we can have the same kind of thing developing down the line, we should avoid this frustration or antithesis or whatever you may call it.'

In fact, this statement represents almost an anticipation that such disaffection may occur. The line structure has been developed partly to deal with it. The implication is that the intermediate level, secure in their loyalty, should be able to impart the same attitude to the lower ranks. In fact, as has been shown, the intermediate level, that is the second group, transmits not merely loyalty, but also the frustration which they themselves experience. Clearly, it would be out of the question for the chief executive to be equally available to all, no matter how junior, and thus this situation does not imply criticism of him. Equally, however, he is aware, at least at an unconscious level, that the situation may lead to a degree of frustration and resentment, and thus create ambivalence among some members of his staff. To accept this consciously may represent too painful an experience. He, therefore, defends himself against this by making excuses for 'these young men'; second, by relying on 'the line' to transmit the necessary loyalties; and, finally, by refusing to accept that the situation does exist. It may be noted that, like every conflict, this ambivalence gives rise to anxiety. This unconscious anxiety, like the anxiety consciously created at times in the sales department (see page 83), serves the purpose of spurring the staff on to greater efforts in order to relieve it and to satisfy their boss. Finally, it should be noted that the chief executive of the company impresses to a very real degree his personality, his attitudes, and his aims upon his organization. The extent of this effect naturally varies in accordance with the individual's own personality and the external conditions prevailing.

One of the causes of this flexibility is the difference of attitude between Alexander and Joseph. It has been shown earlier that at least at a surface level the two men expressed different attitudes towards household products. Whereas Alexander saw them largely in emotional terms, Joseph expressed his attitude by using a simple business definition (see page 99). In discussion with lower level executives there was an interesting and curious attempt to hold on to the two reactions, often keeping them apart, or at least not too well integrated. The following are a few of the replies received from lower level executives to the question: 'What do household products really mean, what do they stand for?'

'[Products B] and [products C] are capital goods. Research shows that the ordinary consumer takes twelve months to make a buying decision. At the moment we ride on the crest of enthusiasm or shall we call it hysteria. How much longer will this hysteria last? I say [household products] are an investment to keep a household running more rationally.'

'[Household products] give a useful and basic service. Now more consumers have become aware of the need for them, for instance [products B]. It is a highly saleable and

114

promotable product, as yet insufficiently and inadequately exploited.'

'The kitchen is the hub of the home. [Household products] afford the housewife more time. They have snob value but they also are a benefit to health. They make shopping easier. Maybe they have more of them elsewhere but the [national] focal point is the home. And less housework makes for more enjoyable weekends with the husband at home.'

'A [household product] is a necessity and not a luxury. It is labour saving and an expression of a higher living standard . . . but keeping up with the Joneses is merely a levelling process.'

'A [household product] represents a relief from chores in a classless way. It provides a happier, easier life, after dusting, washing by hand. The housewife is quick to appreciate features. But the decision to purchase is related to the woman's relationship to her family. The husband still controls the purse strings although the wife may be working.'

Every one of these quotations reveals to some extent a split in the attitude of the speaker. The first one, for example, refers to enthusiasm for household products as hysteria – an obviously highly unfavourable attitude. In the next sentence, however, he is describing them as an 'investment to keep a household running more rationally'. There is nothing of the speaker's in these remarks, only an attempt to identify with the imperfectly understood attitudes of one or the other of the two company heads.

(b) The Sales Department

Twenty men out of a sales force of sixty-seven were interviewed, and evidence from these interviews suggests that the sales group, like the marketing group, can be divided into three broad categories. From a chronological point of view the division is simply between those who were with the company before the new management took over and those who arrived later. However, among those who were with the company prior to the new management, there is also a division into two distinct groups. The dividing line for this split appears to some extent to be a matter of age, with the middle forties providing the point of separation.

There is, however, also a marked psychological difference between these two latter groups. Of the older salesmen who might be termed the 'unreconstructed' group, eleven men were interviewed. They were very reminiscent in their attitudes of the non-leader salesmen, described in Chapter IV. Like them they sell primarily their own personality. Their sales calls have the flavour of social and personal visits, as does their conversation with the buyer. Only almost at the end of their visit, when they have sold themselves and been accepted, do they permit themselves to ask whether the buyer may need some of our products? Even then they do not offer their products, but merely inquire whether the buyer 'may need them'.

Psychologically their main characteristic seems to be insecurity. Therefore, what they are seeking is acceptance of themselves and also of the company with which they are identified. If they receive an order, it represents to them acceptance and they feel elated. If the buyer is rude or critical of the company or the product, or praises its competitors, this type of salesman becomes apologetic and may even grumble about his own company. In the course of the field work of this study, the author went out on call with a number of this group. In addition he held discussions with others, attended sales meetings and conferences, and visited local branch sales offices. During this time the author heard criticisms of the company from these men. It seemed to the author, when he visited buyers with the salesmen, that they behaved towards the buyers as if they were persons in authority and as if they were often reproving them. Strikingly, no criticisms of buyers were voiced by this group, although they might have been an obvious target. It is characteristic of many members of this group of salesmen that they are pessimistic about their own prospects in the company's service, and openly admit to counting the years until their retirement. Significantly, one of these men mentioned this in connection with an optimistic forecast that in the next five years the business of the company would double, possibly quadruple. The author had the impression that thinking of retirement in this context implied: 'Do it without me. This is too much.'

There was evidence of anxiety about the introduction of incentive schemes. At one sales conference there was an attack on the offer of a cigarette lighter worth the equivalent of $7.00 as a prize for the most successful salesman. This was described as a bribe and a 'reflection on their loyalty' proved over a long period of years. In the face of such anxiety the prize was felt as an attack against a method of selling well-established in this group and one which has been the basis of their life's work. In defence against this anxiety the prize is turned into an insult.

The other group consists of men who, although they have been with the company for a number of years and started under the old divisional management, have succeeded in adjusting their attitudes to the methods of the management to a considerable degree. Of these, six were interviewed. Their average age is lower than that of the first group, and their outlook markedly optimistic. Some even feel that the new management has released them from frustration experienced in the past. This was expressed in statements such as·

117

'These advertisement campaigns – I have been asking for this for years. Now, finally, it has come.'

'I'd much rather sell 28,000 [products B] to housewives and make their lot easier than sell one [heavy industrial unit] which may or may not help them.'

'Now youth is an asset and not a drawback as it was before under the [previous] management.'

'Life is more hectic now. Financially, we are better off. There is more pride in the company. Before, the vast majority was sitting on the fence. Now each man has a sense of urgency.'

In spite of their comparative contentment and, even, enthusiasm, they are still fairly distinct from the salesmen recruited under the new régime, of whom three were interviewed. This group, not surprisingly, has no doubt or criticism of the new selling method. These men follow sales instructions to the letter and their sales calls are devoted to active selling of the product. Their attitude to the buyer is friendly but without any deeper personal involvement.

As far as the management of the sales department is concerned, three characteristics can be discerned. The first is a feeling that the success of the company had come about almost in spite of the original sales force, that the marketing and advertising were sufficiently good to cause orders to come in, in any case. One executive said:

'At first the salesmen's attitude to the [new] management was negative. But would they not have worked at all, the demonstrators would have sold the stuff. Now, many of the older men are still in a rut; the younger ones just sell.'

It has already been pointed out that the new management uses anxiety as an incentive to greater sales efforts. When discussing this feature with a number of sales executives, they stressed repeatedly that the salesmen 'brought it on themselves'. By this they meant in psychological terms that the religion of their working community, i.e. Universal, is the modern marketing method. If the salesmen accepted and believed it, all would be well, i.e. they would fulfil their targets. It is, however, only the salesmen's attitude towards this new religion, i.e. their heresy, that prevents them from being successful. In spite of stating that anxiety helps in performance, the executives are vehement in denying that they themselves cause it in the salesmen. According to these executives, they call the salesman in, and, because he knows that his performance has been inadequate, he is anxious. The 'sin', however, appears to be not so much lack of performance, as lack of faith in the marketing principle. This puts the unfortunate salesman practically in the position of a heretic who lacks the faith that would save him. In this ruthless benevolence there is a hint of the Inquisition. There are a series of interviews at which the salesman is given the opportunity of acquiring the 'new religion'. If he fails, and unless he has the protection of very long service with the company, he is in danger of being 'fired' or transferred.

Even among the sales management, however, there is an awareness that the status of their department is not as high as they would wish it to be. As one of them facetiously said at a sales conference held in one of the boardrooms of the parent company: 'They let us use this boardroom here. I suppose, in a boardroom you get wine when you ring the bell. But we get tea.'

Beneath the humour there was a tone of complaint about inferior status.

THE PSYCHOLOGY OF THE UNIVERSAL MANAGEMENT TEAM

In the preceding pages the attitudes of Universal's managers to their business and to the people with whom they are in contact in the course of their daily work have been described, often in the form of direct quotations to convey some of the atmosphere these men created in their work situation.

The author was also afforded the opportunity to discuss the attitudes of nearly all the senior executives to their personal backgrounds. In the senior ranks of the division there were forty-one executives, including the chief executive and his deputy. Of these thirty-two co-operated fully during extended interviews. Some, however, declined to be interviewed; others revealed a hostility that made it desirable to terminate the interviews. Of the thirty-two who co-operated, twenty had come to the company since 1956, and twelve were of long-term service. Detailed inquiries were made of all thirty-two men concerning their personal backgrounds and, in particular, their childhood. Of the twenty new-style executives it was found that no less than fifteen described their backgrounds in a remarkably similar way. Of the twelve men with long-term service only one was found to fit that pattern.

The typical pattern revealed was this: a father often absent, ineffective, and apparently not loved by the son; the mother all-important to him and very hard-working. In most cases, the family appears to have been in straitened circumstances during the subject's early childhood and in some cases into his adolescence. The mother was often said to have suffered from poor health as a result of underprivileged conditions. She was usually described as religious and invariably understanding and loving of the son. A number of these men were brought up as members of the same 'low' church.

120

The other sixteen executives interviewed, five with the company since 1956 and eleven of long-term service, did not fit this pattern. In fact, their backgrounds were so varied that this group was not marked by a common pattern of developmental factors. It should be stressed in this context that it is not the presence or absence of a single factor in any individual case that is significant but the pattern or combination of a number of similar factors that is revealing. Equally, while such views of one's own family background are invariably highly emotionally tinged and subject to distortion, nevertheless, so far as the overt facts were concerned, e.g. the early death or the low status of the father, objective data were often given to support the emotional attitudes.

When the thirty-two interviewed executives are divided in accordance with their length of service with Universal and their adherence to the developmental background pattern just described, a grouping as shown in *Table 3* emerges.

TABLE 3. UNIVERSAL EXECUTIVES INTERVIEWED AND CO-OPERATING IN THE STUDY

| | Employed with the Company | | |
	Since 1956	Long-term service	Total
Developmental background as described above	15	1	16
Not adhering to this pattern	5	11	16
Total	20	12	32

$(X^2 = 12 \cdot 8, \ p < \cdot 001)$

A statistical analysis shows that the two groups differ from each other significantly. If membership of the new-style or of the long-term service group is generally indicative of greater or lesser effectiveness in dealing with consumer goods, the statistical significance of these figures would indicate that there is a relationship between a particular developmental background and an ability to be successful in the present-day consumer goods market. It is quite true that in coming into Universal Alexander has given its affairs a new direction, stressing the importance of the product from the consumer's point of view and in general making a sustained effort to woo the consumer. This, as has been shown, has greatly contributed to the company's success. The question now arises why he and his team in particular did this, when so many others in the industry did not. No doubt, it is possible to say that the introduction of a new management team gave the company's affairs a new impulse. This is, of course, true but it explains very little. In the same time-period as that during which this study was carried out, one of the non-leader companies had changed its household product division management three times without, however, effecting any appreciable improvement in its trading position. The problem that must be assayed is: With external conditions equal for all competitors, what are the factors in the personality of the new Universal team that made for its success? Psycho-analytic theory suggests that the dynamics described in the following paragraphs may underlie the performances and behaviour which have been observed in the course of this study.

Two *caveats* have to be entered here. It is clearly impossible to claim any general validity outside this specific company. Even here, as stated before, only thirty-two men out of a total of forty-one were interviewed. Yet the figures in *Table 3* are unlikely to be the result of pure chance. Moreover, it is noteworthy that, when a draft of this book was circulated among Universal executives, three new-style members who had not been interviewed told the author that their backgrounds tallied very closely with that described in *Table 4*.

Second, the explanation set out below is in part based on psycho-analytic theory. It must be stressed in this connection that a prolonged psycho-analytic study of the individuals discussed here was not carried out. Indeed it would have been very difficult, since, as is well known, such a study would take a very long period of time. In the circumstances, therefore, the psycho-analytic part of the hypothesis cannot be put forward as conclusively proved but merely as tending to throw light on facts that otherwise would remain, at least in part, obscure.

Table 4 presents the salient features of the personal

TABLE 4. SALIENT FEATURES OF PERSONAL HISTORIES OF SIXTEEN UNIVERSAL EXECUTIVES

Father		Family	Mother					Son
Ineffective, absent	Apparently unloved	In straitened circumstances	Hard-working	Poor health	Religious	Loving	Understanding	Attended university
x	x	x			x	x	x	x
x	x	x	x			x	x	x
x		x		x	x	x	x	x
x	x	x	x			x		x
x	x	x				x	x	x
		x			x	x	x	x
		x	x			x	x	
		x		x		x	x	
x	x	x	x			x	ẍ	x
x				x	x		x	x
		x			x	x	x	
x	x	x			x	x		x
		x			x	x	x	x
x	x	x	x			x		
		x		x	x	x	x	x
x		x	x		x	x	x	x

background of sixteen men who have closely similar child-hood experiences. To preserve anonymity the cases are presented in a randomized order and religious identification is not shown. For the same reason the single long-term executive in this group has not been separated from the new-style executives.

It will be seen that the table summarizes a series of perceptions about important biologically related figures, i.e. the son and his parents. Whatever the objective facts of the background of these executives may have been, the perceptions of these men about those figures are important in determining the interrelationship of the different parts of their personalities. Psycho-analytic theory provides manifold evidence that such patterns are formed in the early stages of life and are likely to persist basically unchanged.

Moreover, Freud (1922) called a psychological group

'. . . a collection of individuals who have introduced the same person into their super-ego, and on the basis of this common factor have identified themselves with one another in their ego. This naturally holds only for groups who have a leader.'

Discussing group relationships and the individual, he remarked:

'The group leader represents to each group member a parental figure, while the other group members come to have the emotional significance of siblings. It is in this way that the emotional attitudes evolved in the course of the family living are subject to transfer in varying degrees to subsequent group relationships.'

It is useful, in the light of this view, to consider the attitudes of the group around Alexander. To start with, there is some awareness of unconscious forces among those involved in the situation. The author had noted a marked reluctance on the part of the majority of members of this group to talk about their mothers (only two of the sixteen mentioned their mothers without further probing). When this fact was pointed out to one of the group, he spontaneously said:

'Don't you know that we all have a father complex? We have a big father, the Chairman, and a little one, Alexander. This is why no one mentions their mothers in the interviews.'

This remark, though made in a jocular way, nevertheless deserves to be taken seriously as supplying a clue to the underlying psychology of the situation. It is important to consider how far, and in what manner, these men, while consciously collaborating in selling domestic products to housewives, were at the same time unconsciously colluding in an attempt at a particular shared resolution of the Oedipal situation. This situation can be seen at its simplest in the case of the male child whose love for his mother leads to wishes to possess her exclusively and hence to hatred for the father and wishes to kill him. These in turn lead to guilt and fear of reprisals, which then cause the need for reparation. The child seeks to atone to the parents for the disturbing thoughts and fantasies he has harboured against them. In his imagination, the son has inflicted damage upon the father through jealousy, and has also felt resentment towards his mother for sharing her love with father.

There is in many instances a further complication and a further cause for guilt. Just as the son wishes to replace the father and thus monopolize the mother's affection, so may he feel equally jealous of the mother, who is, after all, the chief recipient of his father's love. This is a desire that causes not only guilt but also confusion and anxiety about whom he should imitate and what role he should adopt.

125

The general importance of the Oedipus complex, moreover, is that, though spoken of in terms of the male *child*, it can, nevertheless remain a powerful determinant of adult behaviour in the persisting unconscious part of the self. To the extent to which an ineffective resolution persists, difficulties will be experienced in later life in coping with reality situations where these become involved with the areas of the personality still locked in conflict. For example, in so far as the Oedipal conflict has not been resolved sufficiently to allow both parents to be loved with relative freedom, then every step forward taken by the man in serving the mother – or mother-substitutes – or in demonstrating his maturity and skill, e.g. in running a successful business, may be accompanied by a correlated feeling of triumph over the father and hence increased fear of massive retaliation. In some cases when the individual has achieved great success, feelings of guilt may become so strong at times that he is impelled in effect to destroy his own work, and bring on failure. That is to say that objective reality-based success, which might be expected rationally to lead to increased confidence, can lead instead to increased insecurity, unbearable anxiety, and, indeed, failure. Such an instance is when a prudent and successful course of action is interrupted by decisions which seem inexplicable on rational business grounds and which can be understood only in terms of self-induced punishment.

In the immediate case under discussion persistent endeavour can be seen as designed to show the parents how worthy the son is. It must be remembered, as far as this group is concerned, that the mother was kind, loving, and understanding towards the son, whereas the father is pictured as ineffective and apparently little loved. In the son's eyes the father, by being ineffectual, has caused suffering to the mother. Thus the son's first objective is, through

126

his worthiness, to compensate the mother for the deprivation and suffering she has undergone. Simultaneously, through his success, i.e. worthiness, he demonstrates to both his parents that he is better equipped than father for father's role.

In varying degrees there is in every man a 'little-boy' part representing more childish attitudes and feelings. The problem, however, is: to what extent is this 'little boy' integrated with the adult part into the total personality? That is to say, how well aware is the individual in his thoughts and actions of what comes from his 'little-boy' part and what from the adult part? If insight is inadequate then achievements of the adult part of the self may be felt to be permeated by the 'little boy' and hence arouse insecurity with the fear of sudden *dénouement*, even though objectively there may be no grounds for this. In this sense, apparent confidence may tend to take on the character of over-optimism, brashness, and boasting, with an underlying fear of a sudden revelation of incompetence with disastrous results. This would relate a fear of success not only to guilt, but also to the danger of abandonment by the adult, as though he would call the bluff of the 'little boy'. This, then, gives the entire operation, in addition to its reality value, also the character of play. It is as if these boys go out together, telling each other they are soldiers, generals, pirates, tycoons – all very potent. But what if they convince someone and he believes them? Then the adult will leave, accepting their competence, and the boys will have to face life by themselves.

This, then, would apply internally to the adult part of the self. There would be no one left inside the self to protect, look after, and keep from harm the real achievements. Reliance would then be placed upon the gang, with the peril that, at the first sign of real danger needing to be dealt with by an adult, all the boys accuse each other of childish-

127

ness, and the gang tends to break up in a chorus of mutual recrimination.

That kind of group works well as long as everything goes well. But, having internally made father helpless and ineffective, they find, when things go wrong, that there is no friendly father there within themselves to hold the fort and see the situation through. There is instead a pattern of sudden *dénouement*, sudden loss of confidence, of desertion, a quest to place reliance on a new leader who, potentially, will also be disappointing.

To put it another way, so far as the motivation of these men was simply to make the lot of the housewife easier and hence in a symbolic way to express love and gratitude to the mother, then, in this aspect, all goes well. However, so far as at least part of the motivation arises from contempt and hatred of the father and a wish to denigrate him, fully unconscious though this might be, then this is quite a different story and leads not to confidence but to fear of retaliation from the now deposed father. It also leads to a need for a strong leader to defend against this retaliation. Such a leader, however, would then tend to be experienced not so much as the real father – or father-substitute – strong enough to bear the brunt of childish revolt, wise enough to allow the children to grow up in their own way and with sufficiently firmly established goodness to enable his bad points to be acknowledged, but rather as a grown-up little boy leading the revolt.

Consideration of the data suggests that in some way Alexander was perceived by this group to play the role of leader of their gang. On the one hand there is a remarkable congruence of background with the linking of the loved, hardworking mother with the weak, apparently unloved, and derided father. It must, of course, be stressed that the importance of this does not lie in its objective truth or falsehood as

128

regards the real fathers; it must rather be taken as a series of perceptions throwing light on the psychology of those giving this account and representing a series of relationships subsisting *inside* them. At no time were these men questioned by the firm concerned about their childhood or early backgrounds, either when they were hired or subsequently. Yet they represent an unusual concentration of individuals all marked by close similarity in this respect. They see in Alexander someone like themselves who has succeeded in doing what they would wish to do. And, indeed, on the economic level, he provides them with outstanding opportunities of pursuing a successful business career. Psychologically, he enables them to assert their aggressive and libidinal drives, i.e. he affords them a wide range of opportunities to show their love to the mother and superiority to the father. They demonstrate their worthiness by being successful in business and thereby superseding the father's economic standing. They also compensate the mother for the suffering she endured by making products which are designed to ease the lot of all housewives, who then stand jointly for the mother-figure. Most satisfying of all, by doing this they are able to earn the praise and reward of their leader, who has replaced the 'bad' father of their memories.

But since what they wish to do has its guilty aspect and since this aspect has to be denied, Alexander is not so much *appreciated* as *idealized*. The belief they convey is that he can do no wrong – they refuse to admit that he has made or could make any major mistake. On an occasion when it was clear that something had gone amiss they reasoned that this was solely due to the fact that others had 'misled him', 'lied to him', or 'badly let him down'. At no time could they consider seriously the possibility that it had been his error. Struck by the strength of this insistence and by its unreality, the author on occasions in interviews pointed out that

Alexander, being human, may sometimes be fallible and that the complete conviction prevailing in the group that he is infallible might potentially lead to a let-down or upset. One of the executives answered: 'Well, then, we are safe. Because he just cannot fail badly.'

Clearly, a danger that needs such omnipotent defence must be felt to be very great indeed, and the mounting fear of disaster, although experienced unconsciously, seemed never far away. One executive stressed that the problem of succession in top-level management was urgent because 'What would happen if Alexander gets struck by a bus?' From other conversations it was clear that this event was believed to imply the utter disintegration of the group, experienced as a kind of symbolic punishment for having ventured upon forbidden territory.

The cohesive force binding this group together is made up of the feelings and psychological needs which they share to the highest degree, so that they become identified with each other. Moreover, Alexander, having achieved worthiness through success at a very early age, embodies their ideal and a desired solution to their problem. His needs are experienced as their needs, and there is little doubt that this identity was mutually felt at an unconscious level at the time they were selected for their jobs. Recalling once more the dictum of Freud stated earlier in this section, it is the leader who becomes the group's ego-ideal, i.e. what they would like to be themselves.

The author gained the impression also that the special vocabularies referred to earlier represented a further attempt to bind the group together and to keep outsiders, and danger, out. It is generally accepted that special languages, like slang, originate within a closed group. Their purpose is to supply a type of shorthand to produce effects and to make others the outsiders.

In view of these observations, it is worth while asking finally how it came about that the author, carrying out an avowedly psychological study, met with such a high degree of co-operation from this group. In this connection it must be recalled that the author is, and was known by this group to be, both a businessman and a psychologist. So far as the latter role is concerned, members of the group left him in no doubt as to their views. The typical attitude of executives of the company to psychology was expressed by one who said:

'I am against all this probing of individuals by American psychiatry. Why stir up the mind? Leave it alone. It is the community life which gets lost and should be restored, and not the individual.'

Several important points may be noted in this remark. On the one hand psychiatry – seen as a disturbing process – is referred to as 'American' and thus consigned across the Atlantic. Also there is the denial that the *individual* needs to be restored. Yet the suggestion is strong that it is essentially the individual – the father – who is really felt to be in need of restoration. But what emerged also from this and other communications was the insistence of the group that the author himself was not a psychologist but a businessman and therefore 'practically one of us'. In this role he could be accepted, and his repeated assertions that he was approaching this study as a psychologist were to all intents and purposes ignored.

A word needs to be said here on the vexed question of 'normality' and the relation of unconscious factors to conscious life. It cannot be sufficiently stressed that to suggest that an individual's motivation is his attachment to his mother or his apparent dislike of his father does not imply that there is any departure from the normal in the individual's

131

make-up. Every human being retains in adulthood a range of significant feelings towards his parents, whether they be alive or dead. Indeed, happy is the individual who is able successfully to utilize these feelings as the basis of a successful career. Nor should it be thought that there is a suggestion that the way to success is in reliance on the unconscious. It is difficult, if not impossible, not to project one's personality into one's work. As a result, the degree to which the needs of the individual coincide with those of the organization that employs him is one of the factors that serves to make him better adjusted and enables the organization to grow successfully. However, it must not be thought that there is any suggestion that the way to success is reliance on the unconscious, successful though this course of action may be in the short run. In the long run, however, if the individual projects his personal problems into the social sphere, and tries to work them out through his business life, danger inevitably follows. This is why conscious hard work and planning have been clearly shown to be essential to the Universal team's success. In this respect, this study has done no more than to discuss the unconscious factors that helped to make this effective, and those which may affect the success of the operation.

VI. The case of the Davidson Company

Some of the main differences between the attitudes of executives in the non-leader companies and in Universal will already be apparent. Before, however, going on to make explicit comparisons between them and, further, to give some interpretations of the differences found, it will be helpful to consider the case of the Davidson Company. This presents points of comparison both with the non-leaders and with Universal.

The Davidson Company was actually founded during the time that the research for this study was under way. It has risen to national prominence with great rapidity, having been formed as recently as 1958 with a very small capital. Within this space of time it has achieved a production rate of a large number of units of product B which, if sustained, gives it a share of about 10 per cent of the market. It has a value as a company substantially in excess of the equivalent of three million dollars.

In terms of the individual, it is essentially a one-man business, in the sense that T. Benjamin founded it, built it up, and retains absolute control. His achievement is the more striking in that he did this on an original capital of the equivalent of three hundred dollars and with a background of unsuccessful business ventures. An extended interview with Benjamin, which was recorded, produced the following account of his background.

Benjamin comes from a Jewish working-class family in humble circumstances. His mother, to whom he was deeply devoted, was clearly of a practical cast of mind and the most

133

important figure in the household. She is regarded by him as loving, warm-hearted, and understanding. Of his father he says: 'If you put him in a shop I reckon he'd go bankrupt in about three weeks. Got no idea whatsoever.'

In its essentials, this is apparently a similar psychological situation to that prevailing in the Universal group. Moreover, there is the added and important fact that it was upon his mother's death, in fact on the very day she died, that Benjamin decided to devote himself to the household product business. He had always wanted to be in business, but, as he says: 'Before that, I had no aspirations for brilliance, or anything.'

His business ventures prior to that date were mainly involved with transportation, an activity with a distinctly masculine connotation. Immediately prior to his mother's death he had started a fairly lackadaisical household product venture with another man. Then, in his own words:

'Well, when my mother died, it was a sort of bit of a void at the time. I lost interest in everything and then I got this colossal interest in the [household product] business and it's been since then really that I . . . didn't care what hours I worked, you know. It became a bit of an obsession with me. Because I didn't go out at all and it was something to do to spend my evenings. That was when I really started thinking how it could be operated.'

Essentially, therefore, Benjamin even more pointedly than the Universal group is engaged in building a business that is a monument to his mother. He is producing a product that he sees as lightening the load of every housewife who stands in his mother's place. The answer Benjamin gives to the question 'Who buys your products?' has striking similarities to the reply that Alexander gave. Benjamin states:

134

'Well, it is the woman that rules the home. She fills in the coupon. She puts on the pressure and she gets it. That's how it works. Of some inquiries we had, 935 came in from women and 65 from men. It means that 935 women picked up the paper and filled in the coupon knowing that we were going to come around and really sell to the husband. Once a woman convinces the man that in the long run it will be an enormous saving in bills, he's quite happy to go ahead with it. Because it's only a few [dollars] each week and it's reached the stage where the people of this country can afford it. You get . . . three or four people working in one family and if they all club together to get a [product B], it's nothing to them. It's not so much one man, now, it's the whole family. The daughters, the mother, the husband, they all buy it together.'

In marked contrast to the non-leaders' narrow definition of their markets, Benjamin declares: 'We cater for people . . . We cater for every type of person.'

Asked about the selection of his sales staff, he emphasizes that he prefers outsiders, i.e. formerly not connected with the household product industry. He says:

'We don't pick them, we just advertise in the national press and we've get two thousand. My star salesman that averages twelve [product B] throughout the year was a taxi-driver. He hadn't the vaguest idea how to sell anything. He came along and we trained him . . . when we advertised we had about 1,800 applications for about 30 jobs. . . . We don't need people who come in and say I've sold everything, I'm the best salesman in the world. Right away we can eliminate those . . . I'm not interested. I'd rather have somebody coming out of the Forces or who has done something entirely different because you can train them to your methods.'

Later, he makes it clear that, 'All you teach them is the advantage of buying the [product] direct, as against going into the shop and buying it.'

In other words, it is not instruction in method that is important but that the salesman should be of a similar background or type to Benjamin himself, preferably unassuming, warm-hearted, and with a background of military service in the ranks. There is no doubt that the selection is intuitive. Characteristically, the sales force, consisting of some 180 men, is run by Benjamin's sister, aged about twenty-two. This seems to be a practical example of women being the driving force for men. As he stated before: '. . . it's the woman that rules the home. . . . She puts on the pressure and she gets it. That's how it works.'

As to his personal habits outside work, he describes himself rather puritanically. He says:

'I don't indulge . . . I don't drink and I don't smoke – I don't like night clubs . . . I've got ideas for building this company into an industrial group. You see, I want to increase the thing . . . I take an interest in most of the parts of the business. I know about practically everything . . . At the moment, I couldn't care less about holidays or anything. . . .'

There is one final and interesting point of group identification. Benjamin wears a neat Van Dyke beard so as to 'look older'. It is relevant that a proportion of his staff also wear beards in clear emulation of their boss. It seems as though in the Davidson group the beard plays the same role as the special language at Universal.

The main point, however, is that there are no signs in Benjamin's personality of the tensions and undercurrents which make themselves evident in the case of Alexander's team. They do not obtrude into his warm and positive attitude towards his own mother and towards women in general. There is an absence of over-idealization of the mother. The father, although he had 'got no idea [of business] whatsoever', is regarded with warmth. In general, there does not seem to be any conflict between his conscious and unconscious attitudes in these respects. This is, of course, not to say that Benjamin is conflict-free but that his problems and his methods of resolving them are of a demonstrably different kind from those of the executives at Universal and are likely to lead to less difficulty in relation to the sophisticated task of selling domestic products to the housewife.

VII. Successful and non-leader companies — a comparison of attitudes

The author stated earlier in this book that in his view the understanding of human motivation in work provided a most important key to the understanding of economic growth. Moreover, the ability to perceive a business situation creatively was the most important quality of managers. The quality of this perception, however, depended on the managers' ability to identify with the people in the business situation without experiencing unbearable anxieties. This kind of anxiety invokes defences which then lead to inefficiencies in varying degrees.

It has been shown in this study that describably different attitudes existed in one industry, in two groups of firms, one called leaders, the other non-leaders. Although all companies were in the same business operating with like organizational structures and under like market conditions, their results not only differed markedly, but continued in the same direction through time. Furthermore, the personalities and attitudes of top-level management reflected themselves throughout the hierarchies of their organizations. This was reinforced by the selection process; managements tended to hire in their own image, and employees gravitated towards certain companies because consciously or intuitively they felt in a particular sense 'at home' there. Once in the organization, the prevailing managerial atmosphere demanded of these men a close adherence to the company's philosophy. In short, the attitudes of higher-level management transmitted themselves to the rest of the group and found reinforcement in the daily interactions among themselves and between themselves and the external market forces. Thus changes in the organization's performance had to be initiated at the top and nowhere else.

Previous chapters detailed differences in attitudes of the two groups, leaders and non-leaders, and suggested explanations in terms of deeper-lying psychological factors.

A word of warning, however, is needed at this point. When two individuals or companies or groups of companies are compared, one of which is more successful than the other, there is always a danger of the comparison appearing as a simple contrast between right and wrong, or competence and incompetence. It is liable to seem that one of the courses of action or patterns of motivation is recommended and the other not. The psychologist must explicitly deny any intention to make value judgements or, indeed, the competence to do so. His task is to describe, to understand, and to explain. The detection of a particular motivation underlying a business situation does not mean that others are recommended to think likewise, even if this were possible, which mostly it is not. Moreover, as far as personality psychology is concerned, any study such as this is inevitably a simplification, since it picks out those motivations which are relevant to an understanding of the business situation. The complexity of human nature embraces a multitude of hopes and fears and attitudes of mind. In selecting those relevant to this study the author is not for one moment denying the existence of others. Equally, is it not suggested that one single psychological motivation is the sole or always the most important determinant of business behaviour. This is most important in discussing the pattern common to the non-leader companies. Though elements which go to make up the motivation of their executives may be of a similar nature, their relative strength can vary widely from case to case.

Finally, no claim is made here that these differences in attitudes always cause variation in business performances resulting in their respective market shares and profit positions. It has been noted that non-leader executives, while less successful in the field of household products, displayed substantial success in other markets. By the same token, leader executives successful in the household product business either deliberately stayed away from other fields or did not meet there with desired success. In all instances these men had shown ability and success in some areas of business and not in others.

Consequently, the question arises: why is it that men proved intelligent and capable in some circumstances act in others to their own and their organizations' detriment? It has already been suggested that the answer to this question can be found in the particular psychological values their work has for them. These values will find expression in their attitudes, which in turn will reflect themselves in their work performances. This, then, poses two further questions: one, what causes the particular psychological values; the other, what are the factors in one's psychological make-up that determine the formulation of the psychological values? This leads ultimately to the most important question: from what source do these psychological factors stem?

In this chapter the author will attempt to develop some answers to these questions by further analysing the material gathered in the course of this study. If the interpretations made in this analysis are valid they should point to the direction in which changes in the result of work performances could be effected. At this stage, the main differences between leader and non-leader firms can briefly be summarized as follows:

1. The leaders are through time increasingly successful in terms of market shares and profits, both important

criteria for economic growth. The non-leader firms, although at times experiencing rising total sales turnovers, do not increase their market shares. This indicates that these gains are directly related to an expanding market and not to markedly improved marketing efforts. Moreover, their profits seem to be arrested or in many instances declining.

2. The leaders' marketing performance can be termed dynamic, i.e. going with the needs of the market and often anticipating them. This expresses itself in a decreasing use of intermediate channels of distribution and effective drive towards direct contact with the consumer. Other ways in which this shows itself are an emphasis on *marketable products*, and an avoidance of price increases, thereby enabling the broad working classes to own these household products. There is no particular commitment to resale price maintenance.

By contrast, the non-leader managements convey the impression that their markets have become too dynamic for their conservatively oriented business policies with their emphasis on traditional channels of distribution, an avoidance of direct contact with the consumer, a thinking heavily geared towards *products of a high technical standard* almost independent of the demands of the market, an ambivalence towards the working-class market and a deeply entrenched favouring of resale price maintenance.

3. Co-existing with these differences in attitude towards their market, there are among executives of these two groups of firms differences in attitude towards their own personal backgrounds.

4. The differences towards their markets show themselves predominantly in attitudes towards women and towards the household products.

141

5. The extensive use of market research among the leader firms can be related to a positive marketing orientation and at a deeper level to a loving care for women. The comparative neglect or even absence of market research among the non-leader companies can be related to their product orientation and at a deeper level to a denigration of the market. This appears to be a defence against the denigrated women, who are then feared as retaliatory and hence must be appeased by 'catering'.

6. Leader executives display a drive towards constant expansion. They seem to be impelled by the realization that in business standing still is tantamount to losing ground to those competitors who move ahead. This includes not only competitors within their own industry but all those who compete for the consumers' discretionary expenditures.

The non-leader executives, however, seem to be relatively inert. They do not display an urge to experiment with marketing policies contrary to tradition. While expressing desires to change they neither devise nor implement measures to stem or reverse the tide of failure.

One of the most striking features of the non-leader companies is that, as opposed to other firms selling products to a mass market, they have relegated marketing and market research to a very minor position, if they have them at all. In the case of the big companies concerned, this contrasts particularly sharply with their readiness to invest great sums of money in technological research.

Modern business holds that, if it is to be viable, it is the business of business to obtain a return on the invested capital and to eliminate risks endangering this return. Market research, having the problem correctly focused and formulated, is a means of providing information which, properly evaluated, should result in a marketing policy designed to reduce such risks as far as possible, especially one set of risks – non-acceptance of the product on the part of the consumer. Moreover, intelligent analysis and balanced acceptance of this information should lead to creative growth of the business. To reject market research and to proceed instead on intuition, so far from being a commonsensical approach, has all the earmarks of gambling. The truth of this assertion is witnessed by the fact that these companies experienced over the years repeated failures in the form of small and reducing market shares, and small profits and even losses.

In this context it is worth quoting Barna (1960), who noted that:

'Observation with multi-product firms showed that good divisional management also showed good divisional profits. These, however, are at least in part cancelled out by low returns of other divisions or even losses which then make the average return on invested capital low.'

The same feature was noted in the course of making the present study, though the author has not been permitted to cite the actual figures.

Popular opinion regards gambling as a very widespread phenomenon and the gambler as a rational person, perhaps of weak character, whose aim is to win money without hard work or long delay. This study, however, is not concerned with this type of gambling, nor indeed with the mild 'flutters' that the great majority of the population indulge in from time to time. In this context it is professional or compulsive gambling that provides the parallel.

Sociologically, Merton (1949) explains that:

'Gambling reflects perplexity about social happenings, and a renunciation of any attempt to understand them. In this sense gambling represents a form of protest against the social process, transformed into a kind of superstitious ritual. It is especially stimulated by social disorganization or anomy. . . .'

The relevance of this interpretation in the context of a changing social structure that so distresses these executives is fairly obvious.

Psycho-analytic theory (Bergler, 1943, 1951) lists several criteria for compulsive gambling. If the behaviour of non-leader executives is analysed in the light of these criteria, the conclusion follows that these men act like professional gamblers.

TABLE 5

Psycho-analytic criteria of compulsive gambling	Business behaviour of non-leader executives
1. The gambler making gambling his main occupation habitually takes chances.	1. They devote themselves to a business which they regard as essentially uncertain, and reject the possibility of reducing the area of uncertainty.
2. The gambler stakes not only his own fortune but also those of others.	2. They are staking not only their own success but also the fortunes of their stockholders.
3. The gambler never learns from defeat.	3. Although their business methods do not meet with success, they nevertheless persist in them.
4. Gambling activates childish fantasies of grandeur and megalomania.	4. Grandeur is expressed in the seemingly absolute confidence in the correctness of the decisions of these executives and the success to be expected.*

*This was found displayed in their product-planning and pricing and at the outset of sales campaigns.

5. Gambling represents aggression against parental authority.

5. The aggression against parental authority is expressed when these men refuse to listen to the consumer. They are refusing to listen to their parents, more particularly to their mothers, by saying in effect: 'I don't have to listen to you. I know what is right for you. It is you who won't listen to me, because you don't love me', – words which the mother may well have used towards the child.

6. The gambler, although at times trying to change his ways, always returns to gambling, since unconsciously he seeks the punishment of failure.

6. This behaviour causes anxiety, particularly in viewing the performance of competitors who achieve greater success. To relieve this anxiety the decision is taken to imitate competitors by copying their products or even by hiring market research personnel. In the main they are often retained to assist the work of advertising agents. However, there is often a gap between the picture presented by the advertisement and the actual product or selling method. This has two effects:

(a) It keeps market research at the periphery, i.e. it is used in advertising but not in the product-planning or selling, that is, within the company itself.

(b) It proves that market research is no good, since, not unnaturally, in these circumstances it fails to work.
This brings on despair about

market research or advertising, or both. 'How much does it help sales?' – implying: 'We might as well return to our tried though *not yet* proven methods'. These methods do not bring success in business, i.e. conscious satisfaction, but failure, i.e. unconscious satisfaction through the punishment necessary to atone for the rejection of the parents, particularly the mother.

Another feature of the non-leader policy is that, in many instances, these concerns market a very wide range of products, covering in some instances more than twenty product groups. None of these has a major market share. The reason for this is variously expressed. One company claims to manufacture every product that is made in the industry. Others say they need to be able to offer a wide variety to their dealers. Several non-leader companies admitted that their range had widened because, after failing in one product group, they attempted to succeed in another. This phenomenon has also been noted by Barna (1960), who says: 'The production of too many lines often reflects a fear of taking risks and also a recourse to the economic power of the firm other than its efficiency.'

From the point of view of economics this is a correct and penetrating interpretation. From a psychological point of view, however, this type of diversification implies more than a mere precaution against taking risks. However strong the company, entry into a large number of fields, in none of which it has more than a fingerhold, is bound to increase production cost, lower profits, and, in the end, lead to economic weakening. There are a number of reasons why a new line of product may not always be successful. But to continue trying it out and to keep it in production for many years in the face of almost complete absence of success suggest a strong latent emotional purpose.

It will be remembered that from the beginning the new Universal management team insisted on concentration of effort on a few product groups, the others being eliminated unless 'there were strong and special advantages' in keeping them. Before this, Universal's wide range of products was rationalized as 'a pride in accomplishment' that is having 'the widest range of this industry's products in the world', a claim which, incidentally, more than one non-leader firm asserts.

This insistence on an unreasonably wide range of products can be interpreted at two different levels. Fairly clearly it fits in with the characteristics of compulsive gambling discussed in the previous section. It also represents a fear of being unable to face concentrated competition in any one product group and a realization, although in the main at an unconscious level, that to 'stand and fight' in one chosen field would lead to almost certain defeat. Consequently, the flight from product group to product group without making a firm stand anywhere is in a sense a recognition of the truth of the situation – a fear of failure – although the response to this recognition is characteristically neurotic.

Similar psychological defence mechanisms can be discerned behind the choice of channels of distribution. The non-leaders deplore their dependence on wholesalers and even admit that it may be dangerous in the long run to fail to make direct contact with the retailers to a greater degree than at present. These men realize, or at any rate claim, that the distributive system in which they operate has an adverse effect on even their product planning. They claim that 'there would be no point in making products with perfect consumer satisfaction', since they must accept the prejudice of the distributors. In fact, the succession of dealers, wholesalers, branch depots and distributors has a double function. At a conscious level the job of all these is to promote the companies' products and provide outlets for them. At a deeper level, they provide layers of defence against direct contact with the consumer-housewife. If the first layer of defence, the wholesaler, were to be removed, this would imply closer contact with the retailer, who is only one step removed from those anxiety-arousing people – the housewives. Although consideration of business reality may suggest that closer contact with the retailer would be wise, anxiety tugs in the opposite direction. These executives find themselves in the position of the little boy who wants to run away from home but cannot do so because he is forbidden to cross the road. Of course, the question is: who does the forbidding? To say it is the parent represents a rationalization. At a deeper psychological level it is the executive himself, intent on protecting the 'little-boy' part of his personality, which would be caught out if the adult part were to say: 'Go ahead, show what you can do'.

A different type of defence mechanism can be seen at work in the attitude of non-leader executives towards the advertising agents they employ. It has been noted that Universal regarded its distributors and its advertising agents essentially as just another means of reaching through to the consumer who dominates its efforts. The non-leader executives, as has been seen, have a very different attitude. In accordance with their generally fatalistic state of mind with regard to household products, their basic attitude is one of passivity. They treat the agencies as though they were experts in a kind of magic and sit back and wait for them to perform miracles. They employ the agency to manipulate an otherwise 'unwilling' and 'unappreciative' public, unwilling to appreciate the offerings of their companies. This failure of acceptance on the side of the consumer appears nearly 'incomprehensible' to the engineer, conscious that 'technically I did my best' and that industry-wide 'it [the product] is as good as others have it'. When sales are in accordance with expectations, the advertising agents often receive only grudging acknowledgement and their fees take on the aspect of sacrifices on the altar of appeasement of housewife-consumers whom 'one does not understand'. But when the sales campaign lags behind expectations, the advertising agent loses prestige, and at times he will be exorcized, i.e. fired, as insufficiently effective in the fulfilment of his promises.

As a result of this the advertising campaigns of the non-leader companies tend to be highly ineffective. In some cases there is a repeated emphasis in the advertising on what can perhaps be described as 'snob-appeal', although this has not been shown to be an effective means of selling these products to the mass-market. Essentially, this emphasis results from inability to identify correctly with broad groups of consumers, particularly the working classes, and also from projection of the executives' own feelings on to the consumer. Its weakness as a form of sales approach is perhaps shown best by the immediate success of Davidson's warmly human approach, and also by the inroads switch selling, emphasizing only cheapness, has been able to make into this market. But to say this is not necessarily to pass any judgement on the competence of the advertising agencies concerned. While it may be that the non-leader companies select agencies 'in their own image', that is, of a kind that mirror most closely their own prejudices, it is equally possible that an efficient agency may have to produce ineffective advertising matter in order to satisfy the client who demands it.

This leads to perhaps the most vital single difference in attitude between the successful and the non-leader companies.

Time and again in the course of this study it will have been noted that there was a pronounced attachment on the part of the non-leader executives to a limited market of a high social prestige. One of them went so far as to suggest 'an exclusive line for . . . the middle class'. (See page 50).

It might be tempting to regard the sociological fact of this preoccupation with status as sufficient explanation in itself of the difference in company performance. From this point of view the purpose of a class or status system is to maintain the relative superiority of one group over another[1] – an observation which will probably meet with general acceptance. Lewis and Maude (1953) come closer to the kernel of the problem when they say

'The whole meaning of middle-class incentive will be missed unless we face the fact that . . . the middle-class breadwinner is seeking more than an *absolute* standard of achievement. . . . He seeks a *relative* advantage over certain other groups of people.'

Halbwachs (1958) starting with Sombart's (1929) observation, shows that the bourgeois' aim was to hold their place in life, i.e. a superiority over the lower classes. Moreover, they expected their trade to guarantee this superiority, keeping the same relative social level as their parents and neighbours, and that to which they were accustomed. He goes on to say:

'Things are produced not for consumption but for the sake of production, and consumers are expected to ensure markets for production at its own price because the development of production depends on this.'

The relevance of giving primacy to production in a discussion of class differential is simply that the emphasis on production,

[1] Sociologists have noted that the country in which this study was carried out is notorious for its pronounced class differences.

150

with an insistence on the technical quality of the product regardless of whether it can be marketed or not, serves to assert the social importance of the producer. It also serves effectively to withhold the product from those whom the producer would like to put 'in their proper station'.

An analysis of the social background of non-leader executives shows that many have worked themselves up from the lower middle and even working class. In conversation many of them admitted that they found it difficult to settle into their new social surroundings – evidence of difficulties in emotionally integrating themselves into their environment. There were many signs that they felt uncomfortable among colleagues whose families had social position and who had been better educated. Consequently, these executives feel over-assertive and experience anxiety. They get rid of this emotion by projecting it on to the working-class consumer whom they consider 'too demanding' and who 'does not know his station'. They find support for this among many potential working-class consumers who, when viewing household products, longingly gaze at them but then sadly say: 'This is not for the likes of me.'

There is a further point. When an insecure individual enters a group in which he does not feel altogether at home, he is likely to adopt the prejudices of the group in a stronger and more bigoted form than they are generally held. Thus an executive or technician who has risen from the lower middle class or the floor of the factory in one of the non-leader companies is all the more likely to dissociate himself from his origins by exaggerated scorn. These two considerations suggest the psychological needs underlying what may seem merely a sociological pattern.

It is worth notice at this point that the dominant individuals in the two successful companies discussed are both considered 'outsiders' by their competitors. It is certainly true that they

151

both come from milieux outside the immediate national social stratification. This applies also very largely to the top management of established leader companies. An executive of a non-leader company was quoted as saying:

'Look who is successful in selling [household products] in this country. Americans, Jews, a [foreigner] Quakers. You don't find an honest to goodness [national] in the whole blooming lot.'

There is no doubt that in a sense he is right. It is an extraordinary and suggestive fact how many of the leaders belong either to national or to religious minorities. Of a leading small firm, one managing director is Jewish and the other of foreign extraction. The non-leader executive who counted off his successful competitors by labelling each, quite unconsciously indicated a feature that supports the general hypothesis presented in this book. It may well be that some members of minorities have more intuitive judgement about household products and their true function in the home. This may represent a cultural factor deeply built into their character make-up, and this over generations. Minorities, on the whole, are driven into themselves and into their homes. The centre of these homes is the kitchen where mother reigns. In some of these groups, the father is rarely the hero to be looked up to, a shining example in whom the son can take pride. This is a direct result of the historic fact that these minorities often found themselves severely oppressed. Consequently, the son is apt to experience greater identification with the downtrodden mother. These executives have entered a profession in which they can actually resolve this problem in the course of their work.[1]

When Alexander first came into the industry, the initial re-

[1] The basic suggestion for this interpretation has been made by A. K. Rice to whom the author is indebted for it.

action of many of his competitors' was a prediction of failure. He was an outsider using methods alien to this business. When Universal appeared to show signs of success, they tended to revile him. But as time went by and the new team appeared established in the industry, these men felt compelled to make some attempt at imitation. Advertising expenditure rose sharply; market research was called in; one company changed its management team. So far, however, success has not followed these imitative moves. Surface imitation without changing the basic attitudes and the basic approach to the product and the consumer does not seem to be sufficient.

It is for this reason that this chapter has stressed not the different methods of business operation employed by the various companies, but the attitudes underlying these methods. Instances have been cited where business methods, if based on a surface examination, can be termed alike among the companies described. However, a closer analysis of the operations demonstrates clear differences in approach, attitude, and indeed in results. As in so many situations, it is men who adapt a system or features of a system to suit the needs of their own personalities.

As has been mentioned earlier, the situations studied in this book have been complex both in their economic and in their psychological aspects. Nevertheless, certain important strains can be seen to be of great importance. Economically, the emergence of the working-class market and the concomitant post-war change in the social climate have opened up enormous new potential in the general field of household products. Psychologically, the capacity of businessmen to respond to this new market has been seen to depend upon their attitudes to housewives, and it has been suggested that these in turn depend upon deeper attitudes subsisting within the personality, primarily to the mother and relatedly to the father.

Among the non-leader executives overt attitudes to housewives have been seen to be compounded of bewilderment, fear, and contempt, and devices have been adopted to prevent close contact with and study of the market. Among the group at Universal, by contrast, overt attitudes to the housewife have emerged as showing concern and respect but with evidence too often of some idealization and, importantly, there was evidence that wishes to help the housewife (mother) were combined with wishes to triumph over an apparently unloved and derided father. Hence success in the market has been accompanied by burdensome fear of disintegration and collapse.

Davidson, by contrast, does not seem to be affected by the kind of problems prevailing among the non-leaders or in Universal. There, the author had the impression that the conscious desire to succeed in business and the unconscious meaning of the various phases of this business operation overwhelmingly went in the same direction. Moreover, they were accompanied by a keen business acumen and hard work.

At a deeper and more general psychological level the main theses dealt with in this study can be summarized as follows:

1. There were firms and their members who 'served' objects outside themselves. They depended on them, and hence the attitude to these objects affected their work.

2. Attitudes to these external objects were affected by what they symbolized in the unconscious part of the mind.

3. The firms studied were all in the household product industry, and the products they made and sold were mainly used by housewives.

4. As a result the attitudes of members of the firms to housewives became important.

154

5. These attitudes seemed to be compounded of:

   (*a*) consciously expressed adult attitudes to women as members of the opposite sex; and

   (*b*) unconscious, infantile attitudes in which women stand for the mother and, in a Kleinian[1] sense, the mother's breast.

6. Study of the overtly expressed attitudes on the part of these executives to housewives and to their own backgrounds demonstrated characteristic differences between them. There were particular contrasts between members of leader and of non-leader firms.

7. It was, then, suggested that these differences should be understood in relation to the individual's unconscious, infantile attitudes to housewives, who collectively symbolize the mother.

8. Clinical work has shown that the infant's attitude to the mother's breast is compounded of love and admiration because the breast contains the source of life and protection. But there is also hatred, since, by virtue of possessing qualities vital to the infant's life, the object can also withhold them. There is also envy both of the unique power of the mother and of the relationship between the parents, particularly of the father's capacity to perform functions for the mother that the infant cannot. This can lead to denigration of the father and wishes to replace and triumph over him.

The infant's capacity to be related to a real mother depends on its being able to establish inside itself a representation of this mother and, indeed, it may be that such a representation exists as a preconception before any actual experience of the real mother exists.

[1] This of course, refers to the concepts of Melanie Klein as described by her in numerous publications and summarized recently in *Our Adult World and its Roots in Infancy* (Klein, 1959).

However this may be, the internal relationship may or may not correspond with the characteristics of the mother as she exists in the outside world. But the infant will react to its mother not only by virtue of what she is in fact like, but by virtue of what the internal representation of the mother is like. If, for example, the internal representation is bad, then, the infant may find it difficult at that moment to have a good relationship with the actual mother, however good she might be.

9. This particular combination of attitudes affected the marketing activities:

   (a) *Among non-leaders* –because their hatred for women predominated and led to contempt, fear, and isolation from the market;

   (b) *At Universal* – where the perception of and the wish to serve the mother existed, but were affected by wishes to triumph over the father;

   (c) *At Davidson's* – where neither of these difficulties was apparent, and where the father was given a real place and the mother loved without the complication of major negative attitudes. This permitted freer rein to the existing business acumen in this firm.

When this study was completed, the author made a series of predictions about the further development of the companies here described. They were:

I. Among non-leaders, at least two firms will be broken up into smaller units, some of which might be merged with other companies, while others may continue to operate more independently. The other firms will either support their household product divisions or close them down in accordance with the general economic climate these companies will enjoy. In short, the operation of money-losing household product divisions will continue only if the rest of the organization can afford to carry them for prestige reasons.

II. At Universal, the author envisaged a marked relative diminution of success within approximately three years, because of the deep and unresolved psychological struggle within the group and within the individuals themselves.

III. For Davidson, the author predicted a continued successful operation, provided the accelerated speed with which Benjamin travelled the road from 'rags to riches' did not prove too great a psychological stress for him. This stress was seen in terms of an internal dissociation from his original background.

The actual development in the industry from the time of the completion of the field work to the time of the publication of this study is described later (see pp. 167–8).

VIII. Final implications of this study

This study has examined and attempted to throw into relief a range of factors affecting business success that hitherto have been little studied. It was not intended to convince the reader of the invulnerability of the theses but to present observations and explanations for their causes for a critical examination. We may now go on to consider some of the wider implications of the results reported, from the point of view both of the household product industry and of other areas of business.

Obviously, there is a need for further study to be made in other firms and other industries. Yet simply to leave it at that seems an unsatisfactory solution to the problem. Two practical questions arise: first, since psychological difficulties were clearly preventing companies from enjoying a full business success, could these have been sufficiently resolved to prevent the kind of failure that did in fact occur? Second, are there any generally applicable principles of business success that might be suggested by this study?

With regard to the first question, the experience of Universal is relevant, since this firm did in fact change itself by the introduction of a completely new management team. We shall later examine in more detail this method of change by selection. But supposing this had not been possible or desirable. Would there have been another way? Here we must turn to consider whether there are in fact means by which an individual can change his unconscious psychology, and the methods of psychotherapy and more particularly of deep psycho-analysis may be mentioned in this context.

It is likely, however, that only by extremely intensive psycho-therapy can the unconscious be changed at all. Moreover, methods of psycho-analysis are inevitably both extremely expensive and time-consuming. It may be doubted whether this method is practical on a wide scale or whether it is in any case the province of the firm to engage in business eugenics. We may consider, for example, the kind of emotional insight that would be necessary for many of the non-leader executives to acquire. To start with they would have had to recognize that therapy could help them and thus that in this sense they 'needed' it. It would have meant that these men would have had to become aware in a deep emotional way of their contempt for at least a substantial part of their market. It would have meant their taking full responsibility for their past marketing efforts, accepting that they were not victimized by the market, accepting also that they were indeed so full of derision and hatred towards it that they were unable to appraise the possibilities in the situation. It would have meant, moreover, the realization that these feelings were directed not only towards the market, but also towards their internal objects, and persons in their lives, in particular their own mothers on whom their very existence depended. One must at this point indicate some of the pain and difficulty inevitably involved in a process such as psycho-analysis. Clearly, it is neither easy nor quick and it requires a strong personal motivation to be carried through successfully. Nor is the market likely to wait while the executives of a particular firm go through this process. This, of course, is not to say that individual therapy might not be a practical solution for the person in planning his own career.

Yet suppose that neither solution – in terms of selection or of individual analysis – was adopted? Might it not be possible for sufficient changes to be introduced by straightforward recommendations, such as changing techniques or methods of marketing? In the course of the study one Universal executive did indeed suggest to the author that any other company that cared to study this book could learn from it Universal's 'secret of success' and would be able to apply the lessons learned. Experience both in business and in the field of clinical psychology suggests, however, that such a view is over-optimistic. It implies that motivation is something determined solely on a conscious and intellectual level and that if individuals are told what their difficulties are or what they should do they will find the necessary changes easy to make. But this ignores the possibility either that there may be no desire to change or that the ability to do so may be radically inhibited by deep unconscious factors. By and large it may be suggested, in any case, that where changes are required and inhibiting unconscious factors are not present, then these changes will tend to be undertaken anyway by the individuals concerned.

In this context, it is worth considering another approach which in some ways lies mid-way between the two that have already been considered and for various reasons rejected. Besides the factors pertaining to individual psychology, an important role is played also by the psychology of the group in which the individual finds himself. Even some awareness of the reality of the dynamics of the group situation can be valuable as far as key members of the top management are concerned. Such methods are exemplified in the kind of laboratory training developed by the National Training Laboratory for Group Dynamics in Washington, D.C. Moreover, social scientists at the Menninger Clinic and other institutes have developed other approaches. Argyris (1962) described his work in this direction in a recent publication.

But while methods such as these undoubtedly have a place, the author's view, based on first-hand experience of the situations described in this book, is that the application of methods such as these would not have been sufficient to enable the non-leaders, for example, to bring about within themselves changes of the degree of depth necessary if their relationship to their markets was to be fundamentally altered. What is often not realized is that even the most orthodox business consultant tends to operate in an atmosphere laden with anxiety and hostility. As a rule, consultants are only rarely asked by managers for the purpose of further improving an already successful operation. They are more often called in by a firm that is already experiencing the unwelcome and hard-to-bear indication of failure. The consultant may then become a focus, both of unreasonably idealized hopes that he will, for example, in some way magically change the situation suddenly for the better and, to an equal and opposite degree, of fears that he will manipulate, take over, or drastically change the situation for the worse. Intense feelings such as these will then tend to determine to a great degree whether or not any recommendations that the consultant may make can be taken in and used. A frequent experience of consultants is that their recommendations are not followed, are filed away, encapsulated, or used as a kind of adornment.

If, however, a consultant is aware of the emotional climate in which, inevitably, he is working, he may be in a position to deal in some ways with the difficulties surrounding his task.

We may now consider the kind of consultancy that may be needed if factors such as those described in this volume are found elsewhere. What has been noted in the present study is that the products sold by a firm and the people to whom they were sold had a symbolic value. Similarly, every product on the market has a symbolic value, since for every consciously expressed attitude there is an unconscious correlate. Therefore, to study such a situation effectively, it

161

is necessary to analyse these symbolic values in relation to each firm and to each product individually. A consultant of the kind now being described, a business-psychologist, on being called to a firm in, for example, the household product industry, would have wanted to make an assessment of the household product market in the kind of terms that have emerged in the course of this book. Moreover, although individual psycho-analysis had been regarded as impracticable for many executives, it is likely that such a consultant would himself find it invaluable, as the author has. If a firm and its relationship to the market it serves can be seen in this light, then the strength of the factors involved in individuals in the firm and their approach to the market can be assessed. If negative or inhibiting factors are not too strong, then retraining, change of job definition, or the kind of business counselling developed in the American institutes described above may be useful. If, however, the kind of deep negative motivation experienced, for example, by the non-leaders is found to be present in such a widespread degree, then it is unlikely that counselling or retraining will go very far. It may be that the firm will have basically to reconsider the type of person who alone will be suitable for its organization. For example, this study suggests that to succeed in marketing household products a genuine liking for the consumer, particularly consumer-housewives, is required. Men with an underlying contempt for women and fear of them, who are driven by this fear to relegate women into the kitchen 'where they belong', are unlikely to be suitable to serve in a key position in a firm selling household products – a business with strong feminine overtones. In this way it is possible to build up an account of the kind of psychological make-up of individuals who are more likely to be successful in this kind of market. As well as sheer capacity, which is always necessary, it is essential that the executive should

162

not be embarassed or made too anxious by the implications of this business. The attitude of the successful would rather be that of the man who, while not liking to do the washing-up, nevertheless is prepared to do so because of his feelings of affection for his womenfolk. He would, moreover, in such a situation not act out his anxiety or hatred by subservience or by the kind of transvestism which could be seen in the man who enjoys donning an apron, but would be prepared to allow his masculinity, his engineering and technical knowledge, to come to the housewife's aid in seeking to alleviate her burden. It would also be important that such men should be financially in a position in their own domestic lives to afford these products through which the strength of their love for the woman's role in the household could be expressed.

The above is, of course, only a sketch of factors that would emerge as a guide to establishing criteria for selecting men for the roles of senior executives in a firm marketing household products. More serious study undertaken by a business-psychologist would enable this sketch to be filled out much more and then used as a basis for the replacement and re-selection that would be necessary for a firm to get itself emotionally as well as technically oriented towards its market. It is worth noting that, on the basis simply of interviews carried out by the author, the attitudes that emerged on the part of executives towards their own backgrounds could be shown to differentiate at the level of statistical significance between successful and unsuccessful firms. Clearly, the possibility arises that such interviews and such analysis could be made the basis of a selection procedure. Moreover, it is not the entire organization that would thereby have to be changed. We have seen how attitudes existing in the senior echelons of an organization tend to impress themselves on that organization as a whole. Apart from those who are specially selected by predetermined criteria, as mentioned above, to set the tone of the organization, there will be other, psychologically uncommitted members who will find the adoption of new images and new ways of working possible if they are given the right lead. Given this kind of analysis, a firm might be able, in conjunction with a business-psychologist, to determine and effect changes of a sufficient order to bring it from failure to success, even if such changes involved difficult and painful decisions.

In sum, the main lesson which can be drawn from this study is that, next to external factors, it is men and their motivations, conscious and unconscious, which help to shape the development of a company or an industry. Economies grow because individual companies grow. The management of a company is an important determinant in its rate of growth. One facet of the problem is that at present it is difficult in the extreme to take psychological factors into account when making appointments. One of the main lessons of this study would seem to be that progress in this direction is required. It would not be reasonable to assume that a unique pattern of abilities and psychological factors underlies generally effective marketing leading to economic growth. Indeed, this study has demonstrated that executives with similar patterns achieved different degrees of success in different fields of business. It has further thrown into relief the importance of the psychological make-up of top-level management.

In its entirety, however, the problem can be seen as one of the unity of the organization. That is to say, the way in which the organization, the people it comprises, its trade, its markets, its shareholders, fall into a dynamic unity, and the way in which they use each other for their own purposes, both conscious and unconscious. In this respect, the study has shown that in non-leader companies there was disintegration. Here the work and the underlying purposes of the various groups and individuals did not fit more or less neatly into each other. These executives projected their own personal motives on to their markets. They then found it necessary to defend themselves against these markets. It can be said that these men insisted on maintaining an illusion. As a result they had to defend themselves against anxieties about contradictions between their experiences of and their assumptions about their markets. To do this, they turned as far as possible from reality. Economic strength often afforded them time for the enjoyment of such illusions. Competitive business, however, favours those who do not only relentlessly seek reality out there in the market, but also look clearly and steadily at themselves and their organizations.

The assertion that personality factors may decisively affect business behaviour is a concept not widely accepted. Indeed, many will reject it in strong terms. One reason for this can be found in the observation that business executives, like all men, often do not want insight into themselves. They prefer formulas which will promise success. This, however, does not make such insight less important to the operation of a business. The essential need for a basic integration between the individual and his work, the actual job done and its symbolic value, has been pointed out. It would seem that only if this is accomplished will managers have no fear of contradictions in their business situations but actually seek them, relate them to their problems instead of isolating them, and then come up with innovations useful for their marketing operations.

If marketing is seen as the creation and delivery of a standard of living, this study has deep implications for the analysis of politico-economic problems such as were cited at the beginning of this book. Obviously, it points to further study and the need to take the effects of executives' motivations much more seriously. It may point to a need for professional business-psychologists in this field, perhaps for non-directive therapy, perhaps for career counselling. Indeed, it may point, at least in some instances, to the necessity of making opportunities for deep therapy available to some top-level managers. Holidays, expense accounts, stock options, watching their weight, may well greatly affect happiness and contentment in work. The author, however, seriously doubts whether these measures will suffice to meet the needs of economic growth on a scale of politico-economic importance.

IX. What has happened since

It is nearly two years since the field work of the study described in this book was completed. The household product market underwent certain fluctuations. The year 1962 was experienced mainly in terms of reorganization and re-appraisal, sometimes agonizing. The market failed to stay on an upward trend, and this despite a relaxation of credit in the country. A characteristic was the success of direct selling to consumers and connected with it the attacks on resale price maintenance. Prices, particularly in product group C, dropped dramatically. Private-label brands proliferated and appeared for the first time for many years in the showrooms of the leading retail chain in the country. Most companies tried to stem sagging profits by cuts in overheads and increased internal efficiencies rather than by growth in sales volumes. Advertising expenditure fell, in some product groups by as much as one-quarter to one-third of that of 1961, as manufacturers concentrated on price action in the hope of increasing their share in a market widely accepted as being dull. Discounts to wholesalers and retailers were substantially reduced on a whole range of product groups. Although official cartel agreements do not exist, these changes have been overwhelmingly accepted among manufacturers. There is general talk of the need to merge production capacity within the industry. On the whole, the non-leaders remained non-leaders; the leaders retained their relative positions. There were, however, some noteworthy changes.

One non-leader firm experienced the impact of a new management-ownership. It came about as a result of a

167

business merger. At present this company is undergoing extensive changes in its top-level management, in the rest of its executive hierarchy, in its resources, and in its marketing policies. It is, as yet, too early to judge the real impact of these developments, although in terms of sales, profits, and market shares, at least in one product group, the beginning seems auspicious. Another non-leader company went out of the product group C market as a manufacturer. A third, after an abortive attempt to get into this market with a prestige product, stopped production. A fourth merged with the Davidson Company.

At Universal, the spectacular success experienced earlier has come to a halt. Marketing decisions, apparently logical in terms of the business situation when they were conceived but less so in the light of subsequent implementation, a reversal of attitude on resale price maintenance, persistent denial of the importance of difficulties at the point of sale resulting from product performance, open disaffection among executives at various levels including key positions, can be seen as symptomatic of the situation. There is, however, considerable inherent strength in the organization.

At the Davidson Company success continues. It has expanded further. The firm's activities have profitably extended into other product group markets. Other things remaining equal, it should continue to develop further, possibly at a geometric rate.

Appendix A   Research techniques

Three techniques were employed in the pilot study. These were projective tests such as sentence completion, TAT-type (Murray, 1938) sketches, and Rosenzweig (1945) P–F cartoons; depth-interviews; and finally direct observations, when the researcher accompanied salesmen on their daily rounds, attended business meetings of the companies, or visited dealers without a representative of the companies.

1. PROJECTIVE TECHNIQUES

People are inclined to deny the existence of attitudes, opinions, feelings, or motives in themselves, only to see them too readily in others. They fail to express them for a number of reasons. They may waver in them, be undecided about them, or unaware of them. They may be unable or unwilling to express them. They may even intentionally or unintentionally indicate feelings they actually do not possess (Cobliner, 1951). Psycho-analytically speaking, these attitudes in the individual are 'repressed' or 'suppressed' as the case may be, but reveal themselves when 'projected', i.e. attributed to others. For example, one executive contacted in the course of this study, and found prone to indulge in spirits, repeatedly threatened to dismiss the commissionaire of the firm for 'too often taking one too many'. He found the mote in the commissionaire's eye instead of the beam in his own.

Projection can be facilitated by presentation of devices which by their very nature are vague and indefinite. A situation clearly depicted, verbally or pictorially, with 'little left to the imagination' will generally permit only little projection. But the less structured and less defined the presentation of the situation, the more it will allow the individual to project himself and structure it in his mind. This process will receive further stimulation when a person is requested to draw specific conclusions. The situation itself being inconclusive, will make it necessary for the individual to produce conclusions out of his own mind.

It needs, however, to be emphasized that responses to devices employed in projective techniques should not be considered as productive of conclusive evidence. People are influenced by moods, occurences preceding the presentation of such devices, or even the presentation itself. This may affect the intensity of a response. Responses can fairly well indicate the existence of a feeling. They will not tell much, if anything, about its cause.

(a) *The Sentence Completion Technique*

In the Sentence Completion Technique unfinished sentences are presented to respondents, who are then asked to finish them with whatever comes to their minds first. Relating to the third-person (The relationship between buyer and salesman . . .) or to objects (Household products represent . . .) these incomplete sentences permit even greater projection than if they were structured in the first person (I think that . . .). Eight incomplete sentences presented to forty-three salesmen of non-leader companies, together with their categorized results, are presented in the Appendix B.

(b) *The Thematic Apperception Picture Technique*

The Thematic Apperception Technique is based on the principles of the Thematic Apperception Test (TAT), developed by Murray (1938). Picture cards are presented to respondents, who are asked to tell a story about the picture. In the adapted technique used in the pilot study pictures were shown on cards. They were line-drawn, as in cartoons, and thereby differed from TAT cards, which are fully drawn. The reason for this change was simply economics. When these cards were pre-tested, they proved to elicit relevant material in a satisfactory manner. Seven TAT-type sketches were presented to the same group. The salesmen were asked: 'What is the situation depicted? What are the events that led up to it and what will be the outcome? Describe the feelings, thoughts, characteristics of the people involved.' Copies of three sketches, together with categorized results elicited, appear in Appendices B and C.

2. INTERVIEWS

Interviews with executives, staff members, and dealers were mostly initiated with open-ended questions. By their very nature these could not be answered in one or even a few words. An opening often used was:

'I am interested in the sales of the Company. Please, tell me anything that comes to your mind that is related to the Company, its customers, consumers, yourself, anyone or anything that affects your work.'

At times it became necessary to guide the interviewee. Whenever possible this was done by means of the funnel technique. Excerpts from these interviews appear in the text. Some may sound as though only succinct and relevant parts of the interview were recorded. They may also convey the impression that the material came forth rather easily. In fact, a great deal of material resulted only from protracted probing. The selection of the excerpts was decided by considerations of space. To give an example of the funnel technique, questions would range as follows:

Question 1. What do you think is the sales position of the Company in general?

Question 2. How do you think the Company is doing in the retail market?

Question 3. Do you think the Company has the share of the market that it could have?

Question 4. (If not): What do you think should be done to obtain such a share of the market?

Question 5. There are suggestions that several features of the Company's sales approach should be changed, for instance pricing, merchandising, advertising, sales promotion, styling, incentive schemes, etc. Can you tell me what you think would be best?

An interview guide was prepared. Its purpose was to check possible omission of relevant points. The interviews lasted from forty minutes to three and a half hours. The number of interviews with one person ranged from one to five, depending on the material brought forth, and whether the author thought that checking and rechecking were indicated. The latter course was pursued particularly when the unconscious material evolved from these interviews was found to be in marked contrast to the overt behaviour of the individual.

It was originally intended to number each interview so that the remarks quoted could be fully related to their content. When this was done, however, it was discovered that the consequent grouping together of quotations made it possible for many of the interviewees to be identified by those who knew them. This numbering of interviews, therefore, had to be omitted.

172

3. DIRECT OBSERVATION

An appreciable amount of time was spent accompanying salesmen on their calls on their customers. Several days before each visit, the salesman was requested, in a Yoell (1947A, 1947B, 1952) type 'camera action' interview, to describe in as much detail as possible his working routine from the time he left his house in the morning until the end of his working day. This information was then related to features observed by the author when going with the salesman into the field. Inconsistencies in actual performance, emotional overtones, and emphasis on special features of the salesman-buyer relationship were noted.

Subsequently, the same dealer was visited at least once again without the salesman. Again, changes in information, behaviour, and attitudes of the dealer as compared to previous visits were noted.

The researcher was able to take notes freely during the course of interviews. These notes were often verbatim. Whenever possible entire interviews were wire-recorded. Protracted, though always indirect and gentle, probing was often required in order to gather the necessary material.

Appendix B   Results of projective tests

The following is an incomplete sentence test consisting of eight items. It is presented here as given to forty-three salesmen of non-leader companies, together with its categorized results.

Response Category	Number of respondents
1. THE RELATIONSHIP BETWEEN BUYER AND SALESMAN . . .	
(a) friendship, mutual assistance	31
(b) difficult, complicated	7
(c) others	5
2. FOREIGN-MADE [HOUSEHOLD PRODUCTS] . . .	
(a) a danger, should be kept out	22
(b) inferior	7
(c) not suitable for our market	6
(d) better styled than ours	3
(e) others	5
3. THE SIZE OF RETAIL INVENTORIES . . .	
(a) determines sales, affects orders	34
(b) is important	5
(c) others	4
4. HOUSEHOLD PRODUCTS REPRESENT . . .	
(a) a high standard of living	19
(b) a modern household	17
(c) progress, intelligence	4
(d) others	3

5. THE BEST CUSTOMER FOR HOUSEHOLD
      PRODUCTS . . .
      (a) the middle classes   14
      (b) young people with children   9
      (c) the now prosperous working classes   8
      (d) professionals   8
      (e) others   4

6. THE APPEARANCE OF HOUSEHOLD PRODUCTS . . .
      (a) is good as is   15
      (b) should be improved   14
      (c) should match the kitchen   9
      (d) others   4
      (e) no answer   1

7. WHEN CHOOSING A HOUSEHOLD PRODUCT,
      PEOPLE BUY . . .
      (a) by recommendation, reputation   14
      (b) by advertisements   11
      (c) by price   9
      (d) by brand name   7
      (e) others   2

8. PEOPLE WHO BUY [HOUSEHOLD PRODUCTS] . . .
      (a) live in luxury, are rich   32
      (b) have large families   6
      (c) do not work hard, are lazy   2
      (d) others   3

TAT-type sketches (see Appendix C), were presented to the same group. They were instructed as follows: 'What is the situation depicted? What are the events that led up to it and what will be the outcome? Describe the feelings, thoughts, characteristics of the people involved.' The results were categorized as follows:

Sketch	Response category	Number of respondents
1	(*a*) the salesman will sell	17
	(*b*) the salesman will get an order	9
	(*c*) the buyer will buy	8
	(*d*) business is good	7
	(*e*) others	2
2	(*a*) the buyer will not buy	22
	(*b*) the salesman cannot sell	5
	(*c*) business is terrible, a bad situation	9
	(*d*) the buyer is in trouble	4
	(*e*) others	3
3	(*a*) the salesman will sell	11
	(*b*) the buyer will buy	14
	(*c*) the buyer will not buy	15
	(*d*) others	3

Appendix C   Sketches

Sketch 1

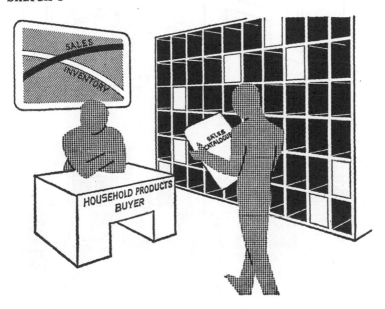

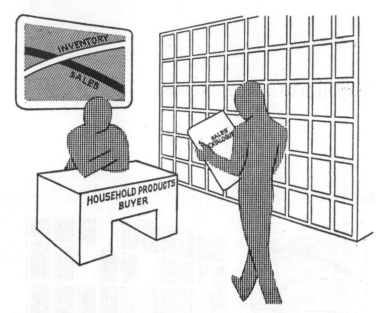

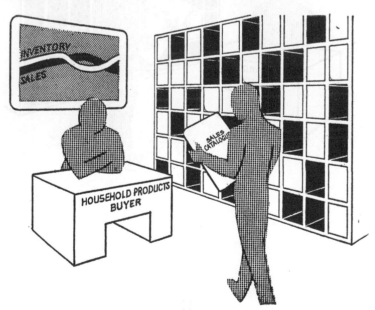

Bibliography

*This bibliography includes only those books
and papers to which reference has been made
in the course of this volume.*

ADLER, MAX K. (1956). *Modern Market Research, a guide for business executives.* London, Crosby Lockwood.

ARGYRIS, CHRIS (1960). *Understanding Organizational Behavior.* Homewood, Ill., Dorsey Press; London, Tavistock Publications.

ARGYRIS, CHRIS (1962). *Interpersonal Competence & Organizational Effectiveness.* Homewood, Ill., Dorsey Press; London, Tavistock Publications.

BARNA, T. (1961). *A Study of Investment of British Industrial Firms.* The National Institute of Economic and Social Research, London.

BARNARD, CHESTER I. (1956). *The Functions of the Executive.* Cambridge, Mass., Harvard University Press.

BARTLETT, F. C. (1932). *Remembering: a study in experimental and social psychology.* Cambridge, University Press.

BERGLER, EDMUND (1943). 'The Gambler: A Misunderstood Neurotic', *Journal of Criminal Psychopathology*, vol. 4, pp. 379–393.

BERGLER, EDMUND (1951). *Money and Emotional Conflicts.* New York, Garden City.

BION, W. R. (1961). *Experiences in Groups.* London, Tavistock Publications; New York, Basic Books.

COBLINER, W. GODFREY (1951). 'On the Place of Projective Tests in Opinion and Attitude Surveys', *Int. J. of Opinion and Attitude Research*, vol. 5, pp. 480–490.

FREUD, SIGMUND (1922). *Group Psychology and the Analysis of the Ego.* London, Hogarth Press.

HALBWACHS, (1958). *The Psychology of Social Class.* London, Heinemann.

179

BIBLIOGRAPHY

KATONA, GEORGE (1951). *Psychological Analysis of Economic Behavior*. New York, McGraw Hill.

KLEIN, MELANIE (1959). *Our Adult World and its Roots in Infancy*. London, Tavistock Publications.

LEWIS, ROY & MAUDE, ANGUS (1953). *The English Middle Classes*. Harmondsworth, Penguin Books (Pelican Book No. 263).

LEWIS, ROY & STEWART, ROSEMARY (1958). *The Boss*. London.

MCNAIR, MALCOLM P. (1961). 'Challenge of the 1960's', Cambridge, Mass., *Harvard Business Review*, September/October.

MERTON, ROBERT K. (1949). 'Social Structure and Anomie', in *Social Theory and Social Structure*. Glencoe, Illinois, The Free Press.

MURRAY, HENRY A. (1938). *Exploration in Personality*. London, New York, Oxford University Press.

ROSENZWEIG, SAUL (1945). 'The Picture Association Method and its Application in a Study of Reactions to Frustration', *J. of Personality*, vol. 14, September.

SOMBART, WERNER (1929). *Der moderne Kapitalismus*. München, Leipzig, Duncker and Humbolt.

STEVENS, S. S. (1951). *Handbook of Experimental Psychology*.

WHYTE, W. H. (1956). *The Organization Man*. New York, Simon & Schuster; London, Cape, 1957.

YOELL, WILLIAM A. (1947A). 'A Technique of Depth Interviewing', *Printers' Ink*, January 31, pp. 33–35.

YOELL, WILLIAM A. (1947B). 'How the Depth Interview Reveals Attitudes to New Products', *Printers' Ink*, February 7, pp. 50–52.

YOELL, WILLIAM A. (1952). 'Make Your Advertising Themes Match Consumer Behaviour', *Printers' Ink*, March 21, pp. 82–87.

180

Index